# MINDFULNESS

## A How-To Guide for Everyone

Publications International, Ltd.

**Written by:** Lisa Brooks and Marie D. Jones

**Photography:** Shutterstock.com

Louis Weber, CEO
Publications International, Ltd.
8140 Lehigh Avenue
Morton Grove, IL 60053

ISBN: 978-1-64030-588-5

Manufactured in China.

8 7 6 5 4 3 2 1

# CONTENTS

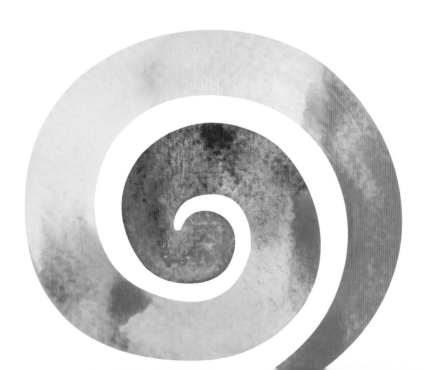

# FIRST, BE MINDFUL

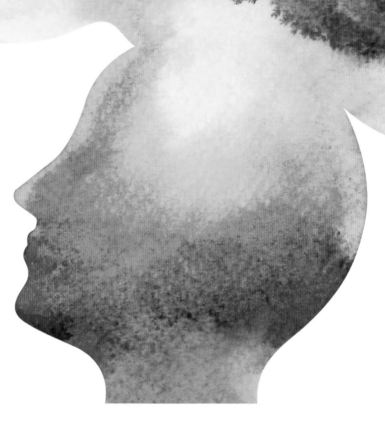

Imagine you are sitting in your car during your usual morning commute. The radio is on, traffic is bad, and you're thinking about the day ahead. Maybe you have a deadline to meet or an important project to work on. Maybe you're worrying about a big meeting or wondering how you'll ask for that raise you've been wanting. Your mind wanders, you grip the steering wheel tightly, and then you absentmindedly reach for your coffee in the cup holder, gulping some down while watching the brake lights of the car in front of you.

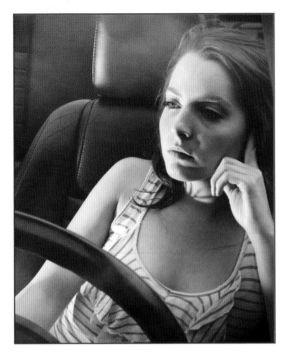

The next day, as you're in your car, sitting in traffic, you switch off the radio. You listen to the silence, or the sound of the car engine, or the sound of your own breathing. You take a deep breath and inhale the aroma of coffee from the mug in the cup holder. You pay attention to your own body language. Are you tense? Are you gripping the steering wheel tightly again? You make note of the colors of the cars around you, and pay attention to the landmarks you pass. Instead of gulping down your coffee, you pick up the mug and take a small sip. You notice the temperature of the hot beverage, and savor the taste. Instead of allowing your mind to fill up with to-dos and worries, you simply focus on the present.

Or maybe your mind wanders to your family. Did the kids remember to take their lunches this morning? Will you have time to make it to that recital this afternoon? Have you made plans for that big anniversary dinner coming up? There's nothing you can do to change anything while you're sitting in the car, yet you continue to worry about things beyond your present control.

By the time you arrive at work, your mind is a swirling jumble of thoughts. You barely even remember the drive from your house. And you certainly don't remember drinking all that coffee.

Now, what if you tried something different on your morning commute?

You've just had a moment of mindfulness.

In the simplest sense, "mindfulness" is paying attention to thoughts, feelings, and surroundings as they occur. In other words, mindfulness is being present in the present. It seems like it should be easy—after all, the only place we can actually live is in the present. The past is gone, never to return; the future is unknown and uncertain. What's more, oftentimes we don't even have control over the situations that cause us anxiety. But this doesn't stop us from spending our days

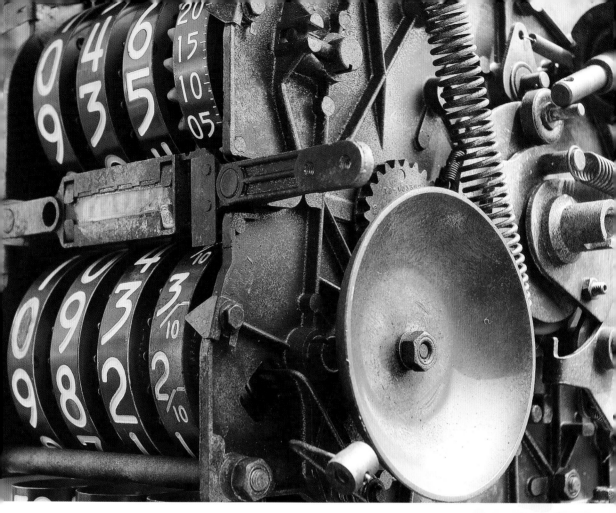

wishing we could build time machines to fix past mistakes or see what the future holds. We allow thoughts of the past and worry about the future to consume our lives. But why? Since we don't live in the past or future, all of this regret, worry, and speculation can be unproductive and cause us undue stress. Making a conscious effort to focus on the present is one way to help alleviate some of this stress. Mindfulness can be a tool to help us live more fulfilled and less anxious lives.

Although it sounds like just a trendy buzzword, mindfulness has been around for millennia. The word "mindfulness" was derived from the word "sati" from the Pali language. Pali is the sacred language of Buddhism, where sati is considered one of the "Seven Factors of Enlightenment." Other Eastern religions, such as Hinduism and Taoism, also embraced the idea of mindfulness long before it made its way to the Western world. In fact, Hindu yogis employed mindfulness in their practice as early as 1500 BC!

By contrast, the practice didn't begin to take hold in Western psychology until the late 1970s. In 1979, a professor at the University of Massachusetts, Jon Kabat-Zinn, created a program called mindfulness-based stress reduction, or MBSR. Kabat-Zinn had studied yoga and meditation with Buddhist teachers, and he was one of the founding members of the Cambridge Zen Center in Cambridge, Massachusetts. He became fascinated by the idea of combining his Buddhist teachings with science-based approaches to reducing stress, anxiety, and worry.

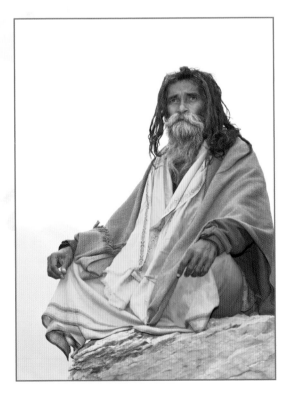

His MBSR program made use of mindfulness methods to help people cope with negative feelings. The program, which consists of an eight-week-long workshop complete with 45 minutes of daily "homework," became so popular that today it is used by hospitals, schools, businesses, and prisons as a way to help people reduce stress and control emotions.

Fortunately, you don't have to attend a long workshop, be a Buddhist monk, or even go to a yoga class to make use of mindfulness. Anyone can use the ideas found in the philosophy, anytime. But perhaps it would help to delve into the basics of the practice before trying it out for yourself. There are several tenets that define the concept of mindfulness, and understanding them is the first step to a calmer mind and a healthier lifestyle.

## FOCUS ON THE PRESENT MOMENT

The main goal of mindfulness is, of course, to focus on the present moment. Easier said than done, right? Sometimes it seems like the thoughts in our heads wander uncontrollably. Almost like our minds have minds of their own! It can take some effort to resist the temptation

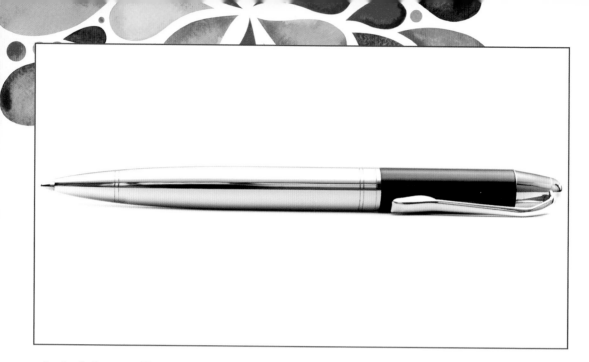

of wistfully recalling past situations or fretting about what the future may hold, but like anything else, mindfulness gets easier the more you practice.

There are two ways that you can focus on the present moment. One is through "concentrated" mindfulness. This is when you focus on one single item or thought at a time, even if it seems inconsequential. "Diffuse" mindfulness, on the other hand, is taking note of your entire surroundings, and paying attention to the thoughts and feelings you have at a single moment. As an example, if you're sitting at a desk, you can focus on a book, keyboard, stapler, or coffee mug. You can even aim your focus at something as simple as a pen. Now look at the item you've chosen and take note of its details. What color is it? When you touch it, does it feel smooth or does it have a texture? How heavy is it when you pick it up? Is it round, square, triangular? It may seem trivial, but by focusing on one single item, you can create a calming, almost meditative state. This is concentrated mindfulness.

Now sit back in your chair and take note of your surroundings: What do you see in your line of vision? What sorts of sounds do you hear? What does your chair feel like? Does it have armrests? How do you feel when you're sitting in it? Is there a window nearby? What does the sky look like right now? How do you feel at this moment? Tired? Hungry? Focusing on everything you see, feel, and think at this one moment is diffuse mindfulness.

Mindfulness can also be categorized as "formal" or "informal." Formal mindfulness is simply meditation. This is probably what comes to mind when most of us first hear the word "mindfulness." We picture calm Buddhist monks meditating in beautiful mountain settings, showing us the epitome of tranquility. Or perhaps you've had a taste of meditation in a yoga class. Even prayer can be considered a form of meditation. It can take a bit of planning to find a quiet location where you won't be interrupted, but formal mindfulness can be quite useful to instill a sense of peace and calm.

But since it's not always practical to find moments of solitude and quiet, many of us don't make use of meditation in our daily lives. When it's difficult to steal away to a quiet location, informal mindfulness can come in handy. Informal mindfulness is having a present awareness of your day-to-day life, no matter what you're doing. You could be driving the kids to school, giving a presentation, or cooking dinner and still find a way to be mindful. You can pay attention to details and feelings throughout the day, living in each moment. Take note of how you feel on your daily commute, what sorts of sights you see, and what sounds

you hear. Think about how you feel when you stand at a podium in front of an audience. Look around the conference room in your office building and take note of details. Savor the experience of cooking, and pay attention to what it sounds like when you chop vegetables or what it smells like when you sauté garlic. All of these are examples of informal mindfulness.

## WILLINGNESS TO ACCEPT EXPERIENCES

Another tenet of mindfulness is the willingness to accept all experiences, including negative experiences. This can be difficult, because we often attempt to avoid negative feelings out of fear. Often, we don't want to find ways to handle things like sadness, anger, and frustration. Instead, we avoid these feelings at all cost. If we avoid our negative feelings, does it change our situation in any way? The answer is almost always no.

There's another danger we face when we're confronted with negativity: If we do allow ourselves to feel negative emotions, there's a risk that we'll get caught up in a spiral of discouragement. When we feel "bad" things, we often feel guilty that we're allowing ourselves to feel that way. Which, ironically, only makes us feel worse! We feel a negative emotion, and then think that it's wrong to feel that way, and then feel even more horrible than we did at the beginning of our thought process. And then the whole spiral repeats, leading to a mire of pessimism or depression.

Although it may seem counterintuitive, when we are mindful, we don't shut out these negative emotions. Rather, we actually allow them to occur, and accept the fact that they are a part of life. We understand that negative experiences are bound to happen. Mindfulness teaches us that not only should we accept our negative thoughts and feelings, but also that it is okay to have negative thoughts and feelings. And when we say that whatever we are thinking and feeling is okay, those emotions lose their power over us. What's more, we are able to understand that we have power over them.

When we realize that we are larger than our emotions, it can empower us to control them more effectively. Some people who practice mindfulness even make use of an unusual exercise where they assign colors, shapes, or textures to their feelings. It may seem a strange concept at first, but by defining emotions in this way— perhaps saying that anger is "red"

or sadness is "blue"—it reinforces the realization that we are larger than our emotions. We accept the "red" or the "blue," but knowing they are simply "colors" helps us to move past them.

## VIEWING FEELINGS IN A NON-JUDGMENTAL WAY

Another important component of practicing mindfulness is perceiving emotions and experiences without judgment. This means that negative emotions should not be considered "bad," and positive emotions should not be considered "good." Rather, when being mindful, emotions are simply accepted. And our reactions to positive or negative emotions should be the same.

For instance, say you're in line at the grocery store, and someone cuts in front of you. Your immediate reaction might be to indignantly argue or to cross your arms in frustration, because this incident has roiled up "bad" feelings of annoyance and irritation. And even if you don't call out the line-cutter on their infraction, chances are you'll feel "bad" emotions about it until you reach the cash register.

But what if you decided to practice mindfulness while you waited in line? When your fellow shopper cut in

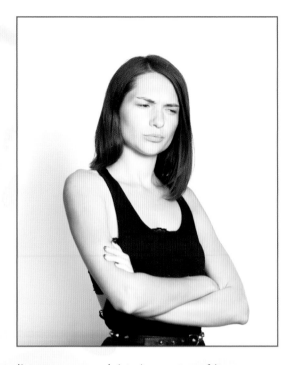

as "good" emotions. But when being mindful, even good emotions should be experienced without judgment. In this way, we can learn to not think of any particular emotion as "good" or "bad," but simply acknowledge that these emotions are part of the human experience.

# ACCEPTANCE OF PRESENT REALITY

Inventor Alexander Graham Bell once said, "When one door closes another door opens; but we so often look so long and so regretfully upon the closed door that we do not see the ones which open for us." Who hasn't looked into the past and wished they could reopen a closed door? How often do we spend too much time regretting past mistakes or hoping for a second chance? Most people are guilty of gazing too long at one of those closed doors, and we probably miss out on new opportunities because of it.

line, you would take note of it, pay attention to how it made you feel, and then perhaps say to yourself, "I feel anger." But instead of reacting in an "angry" way or automatically accepting that anger is "bad," you would look at your anger without judgment. Maybe you would assign a color or texture to your anger, and consider it "red" or perhaps "rough" like sandpaper. By simply accepting your anger and acknowledging it without judging it, you wield power over the emotion and can more easily move on.

But the same goes for positive emotions as well. Just as it is tempting to think of anger and sadness as "bad" emotions, it's easy to consider happiness and gratitude

Longing for the past isn't our only mistake. We also worry about the future. But as President Abraham Lincoln said, "The best thing about the future is that it comes only one day at a time." When so much of our future is uncertain, why do we spend such a large amount of time obsessing over it?

All of our thoughts about the past and future usually end up being a waste of time. There is literally nothing we can do to change the past, but it doesn't stop us from rehashing past mistakes over and over. We might regret things that we've done, or be embarrassed about mistakes, or wish we'd taken chances we never took, but all the ruminating in the world won't change any of it. And although we have a measure of control over our own futures, we only have, as Lincoln stated, "one day at a time" with which to work.

Mindfulness teaches that instead of longing for the past or worrying about the future, we should focus on the present and accept our existing situation. After all, this "one day" is the only day in which we can actually live. Today is the only day we have for making changes, trying new experiences, or taking action. Until someone invents a time machine, yesterday will always be gone and tomorrow will always be out of reach. Dwelling on these inaccessible goals can cause dissatisfaction with wherever we are in our present lives and prompt us to long for something different. But by practicing mindfulness, we can stop the thought processes that cause us distress. Instead of constantly trying to change the present, we accept it for what it is. And it is easier to

accept the present when longings for the past and anxiety about the future don't burden our minds.

## NON-ATTACHMENT

Accepting the present doesn't mean we have to be resigned to live in a stagnant situation for the rest of our lives. Just because we focus on and accept the present doesn't mean we must remain mired in motionless inaction. On the contrary— mindfulness recognizes that life is in a constant state of change. In fact, life changes so much that when we are mindful, we recognize that wherever we are at the present moment is not permanent. We know that our "present" today will

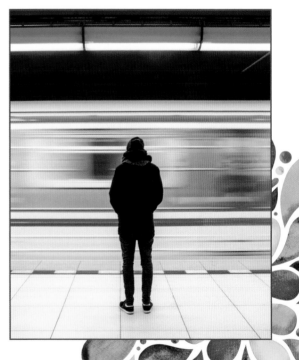

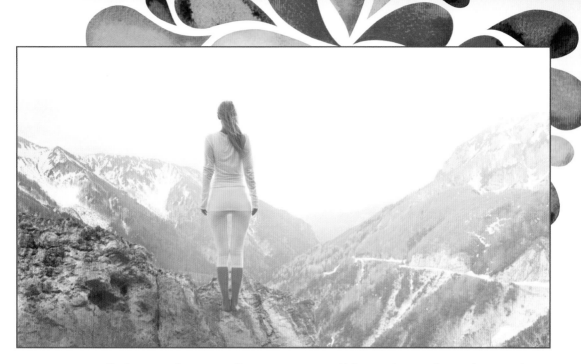

not necessarily be our "present" tomorrow. Because of that, it is important to look at our situations with a sense of non-attachment.

Looking at the present with non-attachment makes the idea of change easier to handle. So while mindfulness does help us to accept our present state of being, it also makes it easier to move forward. It almost seems like an oxymoron in the philosophy of mindfulness. How is it that accepting your present state can make changing your situation easier? The key is knowing that once you have accepted your present, nothing impedes your movement. When you're tied to the wistfulness of the past, or hindered by fears of the future, it can cause a sense of indecision. Once you free yourself from those thoughts and worries, moving forward can actually be an easier process.

Living a mindful life without attachment even welcomes these life changes. Accept today, but realize that things may be completely different in your life next year than they are this year.

## PATIENCE, PEACE, AND TRUST

Finally, approach the practice of mindfulness with an attitude of patience, peace, and trust. Have patience with yourself and with the practice. It can be tempting to want to rush from one thing to the next, especially when our lives are so busy and we have schedules to keep. Although your mind may wander at

# BODY SCANNING

Most of the time, you would be discouraged from lying down during meditation because of the natural tendency to drift off to sleep. However, doing a meditation body scan requires you be in a comfortable supine position so that you can focus your mind on each part of the body while in a totally relaxed state.

You can start with an overall awareness of your body. As you breathe in and out, be aware of areas that feel different or heavier. You are not trying to "heal" these areas but simply become aware of them. Sensations of heaviness at different body points, such as the abdomen or throat, can indicate issues that have not been addressed either physiologically or emotionally, and these sensations may even point to something in the subconscious that is causing you to feel discomfort. Also take note of emotions that arise when your focus sweeps over certain areas of the body. They are trying to tell you something! After performing this overview of the body, you can then start at the tips of your toes and bring total focus and awareness to each specific body part as you move up to the crown of the head.

Because many people fall asleep during body scans, it might be beneficial to use a guided meditation app or audio recording. Listening to someone else's voice can keep you focused. A recording may also prevent you from nodding off in the middle of the scan.

Body scans don't have to take hours. Once you get the hang of it, you can do a scan in a shorter period of time. Identifying the parts of the body that feel askew can help you send a little extra love to those areas. But be aware that the body often acts as a symbol for deeper issues that need to be addressed—like anger, unexpressed grief, resentment, or other suppressed fears. Do your best to understand what the body is trying to communicate.

During body scans, people often report flashes of memories of events from the past that may have traumatized them. If your body is bringing up something and begging it be addressed, you may want to contact a therapist or professional to assist you in processing the event and healing from its aftereffects.

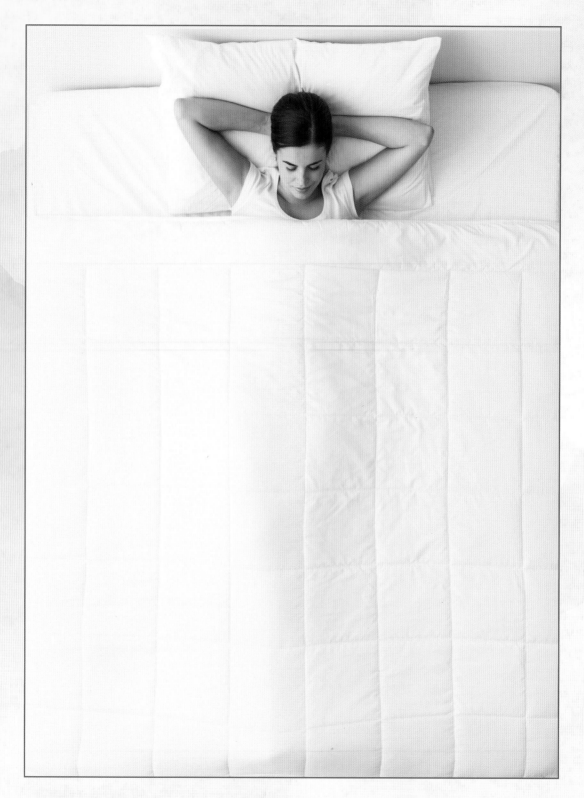

first, with practice, it will be easier to be mindful and maintain focus on the present. Have patience, also, with whatever changes you hope to see. Whether it's a better attitude, a healthier lifestyle, or more motivation, changes don't always appear overnight.

As many of the other tenets suggest, it is also important to practice mindfulness with a sense of peace. After all, it can be difficult to be non-judgmental toward negative feelings if you don't first approach them with a peaceful attitude. Always strive to maintain an even keel, no matter what is happening in your present situation. Things won't always work out the way you

hoped, but a peaceful acceptance of the moment will make it easier to continue moving forward. And trust in your own intuition and feelings while you practice mindfulness. Trust that the changes you are hoping for will occur, in their own time. And trust that you have all the strength and tools that you need within you to live a healthier, more balanced lifestyle.

## READY TO TRY IT OUT?

Now that you have a better understanding of the ideas that form the basis for mindfulness, you can soon try out the practice for yourself. But perhaps, even after reading more about the philosophy, you're still wondering: Why practice this thing called mindfulness? Are there actually any benefits to it? Can it really be beneficial to concentrate on the nuances of a pen, or to take note of my surroundings?

The short answer is: yes!

The ancient practitioners of mindfulness believed it was a way to promote well-being and peace in those who followed the philosophy, and it turns out that modern science supports this assumption. After mindfulness began gaining popularity in the West, people took notice of the effects the practice seemed to have, and their observations were quite enlightening.

When Kabat-Zinn first created his MBSR program, one of the discoveries he made was that the practice of mindfulness helped to alleviate chronic pain in patients with debilitating illnesses. Armed with this interesting and surprising information, scientists began exploring the practice more thoroughly. They noticed that when patients focused on the present and used the tools they learned in the MBSR program, certain areas of their brains were more active. Studies have shown that one of these areas activated during mindfulness is a part of the brain responsible for resilience. This means that when we practice mindfulness, we become more willing to tackle problems head-on, as opposed to hiding from them or running away. Our brains are better able to recognize that we can bounce back from setbacks and keep moving forward. This resilience can be a useful quality to hone in a world with so many ups and downs. After all, how often do we wish we could simply go back to bed and cower under the covers all day instead of facing a difficult issue?

And resilience isn't the only improved function researchers have found. After using MRI machines to scan the brains of people before and after mindfulness sessions, scientists discovered differences in pre-mindful and post-mindful brain activity. After practicing mindfulness, people had more activity in a part of the brain

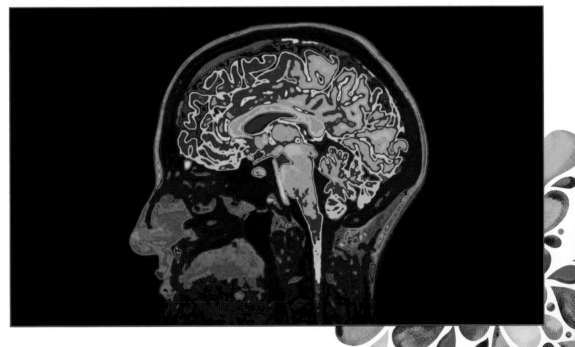

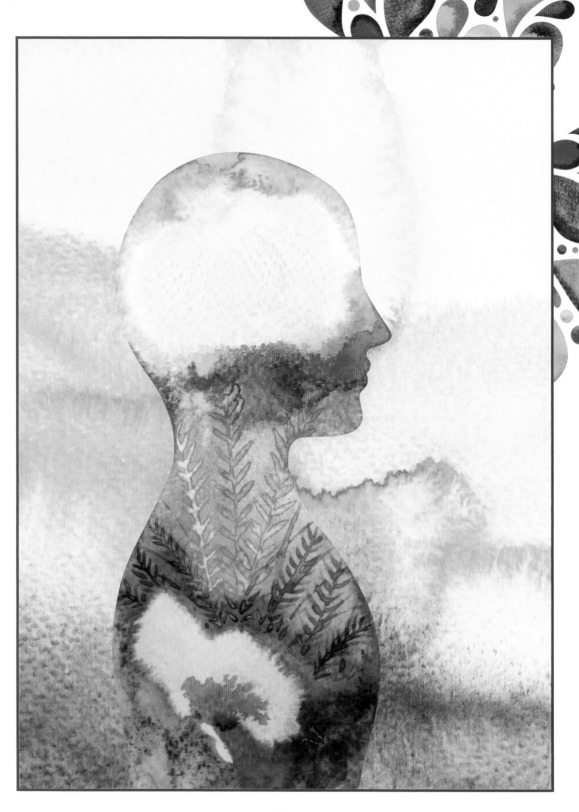

associated with direct sensory experiences, and less activity in a part associated with self-scrutiny. This means people who embrace mindfulness are also more likely to embrace their experiences and less likely to criticize themselves.

For instance, once you begin to practice mindfulness, perhaps you'll see situations in a new light. Instead of berating yourself for a mistake, you can see it as a learning experience and appreciate the lesson. Or maybe instead of worrying about how you look in a swimsuit at the beach, you can focus on how the sun feels on your skin, and how the sand feels between your toes, and what the crashing waves sound like.

Another thing researchers have found is that the "fight or flight" area of the brain actually shrinks after practicing mindfulness—meaning that the body is less likely to have a severe response to stress. So even when life gets hectic, crazy, or tense, you are better able to handle it. You feel less fear when dealing with a stressful situation, and are more easily able to recover from negativity.

But perhaps the most amazing discovery scientists have made about mindfulness is that patients who regularly engage in mindful behavior actually improve their immune systems. A study conducted by the University of California, Los Angeles even concluded that mindfulness practice strengthened the immune systems of patients with the HIV virus. And reported benefits don't stop there—the results of mindfulness are numerous. In addition to providing pain relief, helping to cope with difficult thoughts and situations, and instilling those who practice with feelings of self-acceptance, it has also been shown to lower blood pressure, decrease anxiety and depression, help with addictions, eating disorders, and obsessive-compulsive behavior, and improve focus and concentration. Mindfulness has even been shown to decrease drug use and increase optimism in prison inmates, and

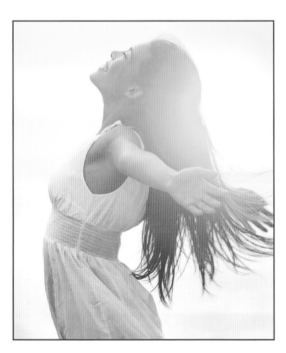

reduce the likelihood of a relapse of criminal behavior.

This is not to say that practicing mindfulness will cure diseases or solve every problem you have, but the science seems to agree that it can provide you with some concrete tools to live a healthier life. All in all, it would seem the benefits of mindfulness are numerous and worthwhile. And it certainly can't hurt to give it a try! So let's look at some more specific examples of how to incorporate mindfulness into our daily lives.

As mentioned, formal and informal are the two types of mindfulness. Formal mindfulness, or mindfulness meditation, can be a great tool to help you prepare for a long day or unwind at night. Try not to worry about any excuses that might pop up. Perhaps you think you won't be able to find the time, or you'll be bored if you meditate, or you won't be able to quiet your mind enough to gain any benefits. You can start with a few minutes a day—anyone can find a few extra minutes in their schedule, right? Don't think of mindfulness meditation as "boring"—think of it as taking some time away from all the pressures and expectations of your normal life. Perhaps you'll find that a few minutes of "boredom" are actually refreshing! And if your mind is

racing, so be it. Remember that the point of mindfulness is to pay attention to the moment—if your mind is full of thoughts and worries at the present moment, simply take note of those thoughts as you practice your meditation.

To start, find a quiet location and a comfortable seat. You can sit in a chair, or just sit on the floor, if you prefer. Begin by focusing on your breathing—the steady "in" and "out" of each breath. If you like, you can focus on a single word, like "calm" or "peace" or any other word that resonates with you. If you have specific goals, you can choose words with more meaning. For example, if you're trying to lose weight, you could focus on words like "strong" or "healthy." If you're striving for less stress and more gratitude in your life, you can think about "happy" or "blessed."

Now pay attention to the way your body feels, and observe any sights or sounds nearby. As you sit quietly, allow your thoughts to come and go, and take note of the emotions each thought conjures up. Remember to observe everything without judgment and to accept your thoughts as they occur. At first, you may find it difficult not to daydream or to not allow yourself to be critical of your thoughts and feelings. But simply redirect your mind back to a place of acceptance and non-judgment when this occurs.

Some experts believe that the most benefit from mindfulness meditation comes from 20 minutes of meditation a day. If that seems like a long time to sit quietly, start with just a few minutes, and work your way up to longer sessions. It may feel awkward at first to practice mindfulness meditation, but with some time and patience, you may find that it becomes an integral part of your daily routine.

But if meditation just isn't your thing, or your day is too busy to squeeze in some solitude, informal mindfulness is something you can still practice—anytime. For informal mindfulness, you don't necessarily need to be in a quiet location, although it may help to have fewer distractions as you get used to the process. For instance, if you're at home, you can turn off the television and put your phone on silent so you're not interrupted by calls or texts. But informal mindfulness can literally occur anywhere—even in crowded, noisy locations like subways or

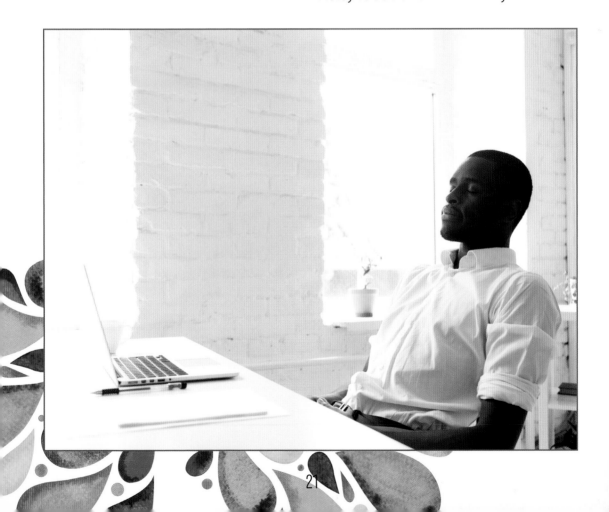

# GUIDED MEDITATIONS

For those who have a difficult time staying focused on their own, there are hundreds of guided meditations available for purchase or for free. Many can be downloaded to tablets, cell phones, and laptops.

Choosing the right meditations comes down to finding a voice and tone that is soothing. It's also important to make sure that any background music, if provided, doesn't irritate you or grate on your brain.

There are guided meditations that keep the mind focused on the present moment using prompts, more complex meditations that go beyond mindfulness and into the realm of an altered state of conscious awareness, and everything in between. Obviously, these are not to be used while driving or working in a situation where it could be dangerous, but a guided meditation can be utilized while walking, hiking, sitting, or even floating in a pool.

Personal tastes will also dictate how "spiritual" you want the guided material to be. You might prefer just having a voice to focus on, or you might like the idea of combining present awareness with postive affirmations and empowering thoughts.

Guided meditations are not the same as guided visualizations, which take you on an interactive journey into realms of the mind. Guided visualizations can involve creating a safe place or sacred location where you can meet with spirit guides, all done for a purpose beyond merely becoming aware and anchored in the present. They are not considered an exercise in mindfulness but are certainly another useful part of a greater spiritual practice.

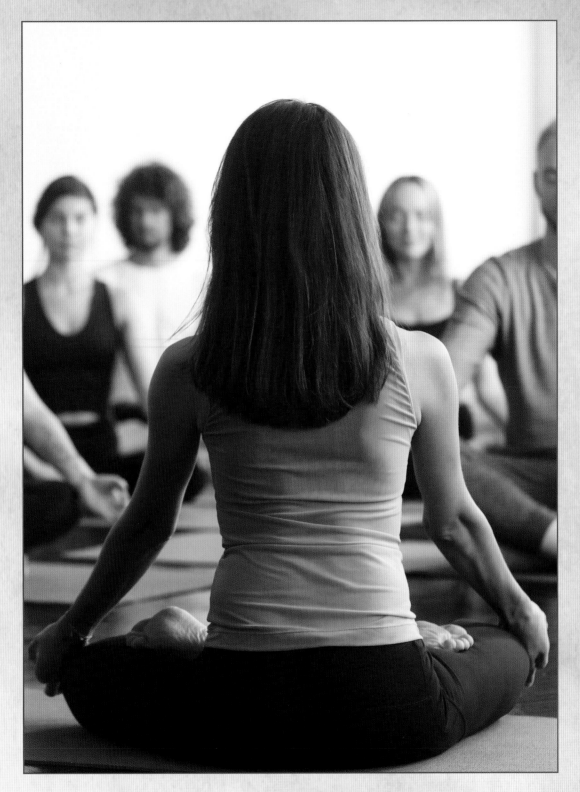

shopping centers. The key is to remember to stay focused on the present, even when things get hectic.

You could spend an entire day aiming for moments of mindfulness, so let's start with your morning wake-up call. Instead of a harsh alarm, try waking up to a favorite song or a less-jarring sound, like chirping birds or a babbling brook. Take note of the sound that woke you up, and pay attention to what your first thoughts are in the morning. How are you feeling?

Content? Still sleepy? Worried about the day ahead? Again, simply take note of your feelings and view them without judgment. Before you get out of bed, take a few deep breaths and pay attention to each one. Stretch your limbs and take note of how your body feels. Once you're out of bed and starting your day, you can even be mindful of mundane things, like brushing your teeth—pay attention to how the brush feels in your mouth, or the minty sensation of the toothpaste. If you have time before running out the door, take some time to slow

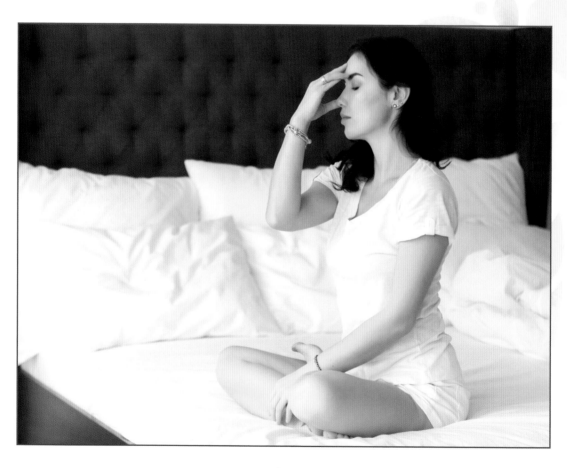

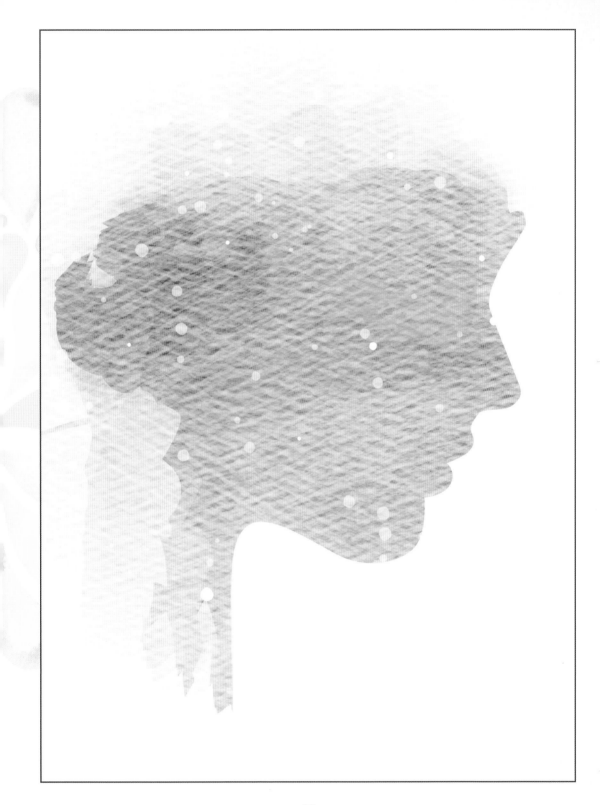

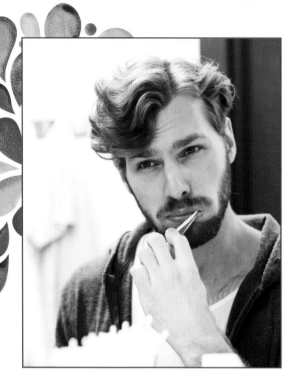

heading into a meeting. Simply take a quick deep breath, or pause to collect your thoughts and focus on your feelings. You can take a few moments before answering emails, as well. Read through each message and then take some time before forming responses. How does each message make you feel? Stressed? Overwhelmed? Appreciated? Undervalued? Whatever emotion is conjured up, accept it without judgment and then continue. This may even help you to approach messages in a less emotional, more professional way throughout the day.

If you're able to, take a walk during lunch, and spend some time in mindful contemplation. If you have green space nearby, take the opportunity to wander through nature, paying attention to the sounds of wind in the trees or chirping birds. Take note of the weather. As you walk, think about how you feel. Maybe the walk makes you feel energized and happy. Or perhaps melancholy and wistful. No matter what you feel, simply take note of it, accept it, and continue with your walk.

Continue practicing mindfulness in these ways throughout your work day and on your commute home, and perhaps you'll discover that you have a calmer, more productive day. Once at home, you can sneak

down and mindfully eat breakfast. Remember the commuting example from the beginning of the chapter? Drive to work without the radio on, observe your surroundings, and take note of your thoughts and feelings before starting your work day.

One way to practice mindfulness throughout the day is by pausing before taking an action. So before you head into the office, take a few minutes to quietly sit at your desk or in your car before tackling the tasks of the day. Take a few deep breaths, take note of the sights and sounds nearby, and allow your thoughts and feelings to come and go. You can also pause in other areas of the day—before answering a ringing phone, for example, or before

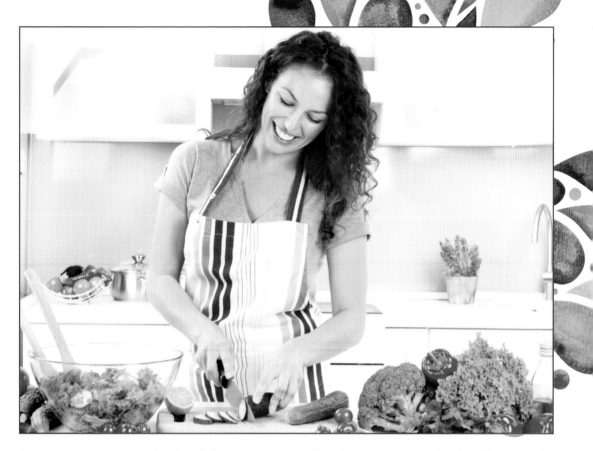

in more moments of mindfulness in between family obligations or distractions. For instance, if you cook dinner, pay extra attention to the process. Take note of the texture of vegetables, and listen to the sound each makes when you chop and slice. And of course, be sure to inhale each smell and aroma of the cooking process.

An entire day of mindfulness is great to strive for, but perhaps your day is nothing like the previous example. What if your day is filled with distractions, like crowded train rides, trips to a noisy grocery store, or family gatherings? It's still possible to practice moments of mindfulness even when our days are packed with activity and commotion. The most important thing is to be aware of your own thoughts and feelings, and to pay attention in the moment. The beauty of informal mindfulness is that it really is about moment-to-moment awareness—even if those moments are chaotic and noisy.

So if, for instance, you're walking down a busy city street, you can still be mindful of the present. Instead of wandering the sidewalk with your phone in your hand, put it away and listen to the city. The noises may be loud or disordered, but take note of what you hear, and appreciate its unique cacophony. Maybe the noise or chaos makes you feel stressed or annoyed. Remember that it's okay to feel emotions that we perceive as "negative." Try not to label them as "bad." Pay attention to what it feels like as your heels strike hard pavement, and notice the cracks or unevenness of surfaces. Look at the architecture of the buildings around you—perhaps you'll notice something you never noticed before. Simply live in the moment, embracing each experience.

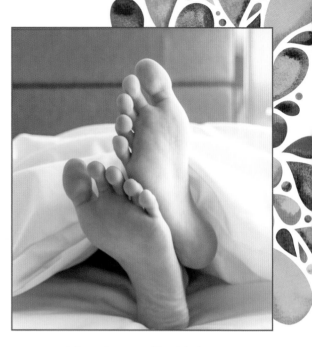

You can even practice mindfulness when you're taking care of kids who need your attention. It can be difficult at first, since you may only have a few seconds to really focus on anything other than the needs of your children. And as a parent, you may feel like your attention is focused on multiple points at once. But you can practice reacting to the stresses of parenting in a mindful way, by taking deep breaths before responding to behavior, and accepting the fact that no parent is "perfect." When mindfulness teaches us to accept our thoughts and feelings, it also helps us realize that it's okay to not be flawless but rather human. As with every other aspect of mindfulness, just try to live in the moment—even if that

moment involves spilled juice or crayon drawings on the walls. Over time, with practice, you may find that it's easier to react calmly to the craziness that is childhood, and you may even be able to pass along some of your mindfulness techniques to your kids as they get older.

So are you ready to add some mindfulness into your life? It doesn't happen automatically—we must take the initiative to be mindful, and make an effort to live in the present and be aware of each moment. But as we've seen, the benefits can be meaningful and worth the work. Now that you're armed with more information, you can strive to be present in the present.

Your mind and body will thank you.

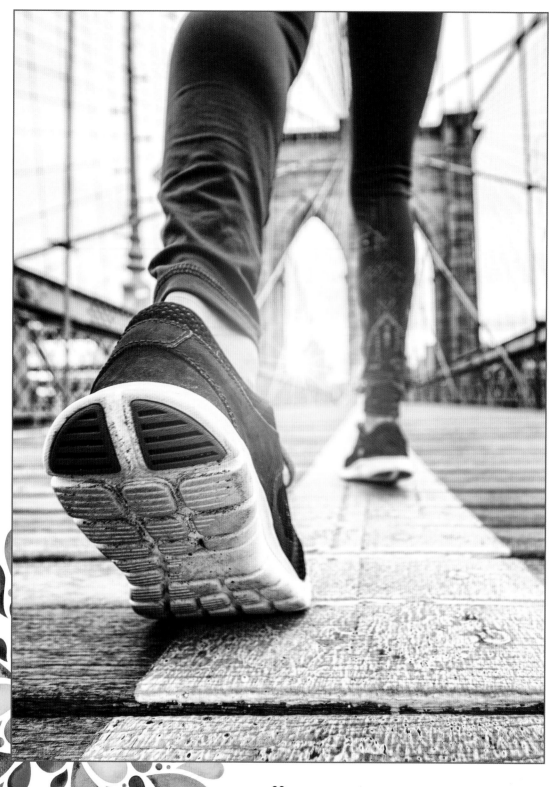

# MANTRAS AND VISUAL AIDS

One way to easily keep the mind focused on the breath is to use a mantra, or "sacred utterance." A mantra is a carefully chosen word or phrase, or a visual item like a burning candle, to keep your awareness right where you want it. Mantras serve as tools that bring a sense of sacredness to your practice. Using a simple and memorable word or phrase that is repeated over and over creates an altered state of consciousness where you become more receptive to the gifts of awareness and wisdom available to you in the present moment.

Mantras are a mainstay of Buddhism, Hinduism, Jainism, and Sikhism. The use of words, phrases, lyrics, chants, and hymns are a part of most religious and spiritual traditions and have more recently become popular with yoga and meditation practices.

Some of the most popular mantras are:

AUM/OM – A powerful sound that vibrates through the whole body and is said to be the first sound heard at the time the universe was created. The mantra is said slowly and deliberately to bring about a sensation of energy moving throughout the body from the pelvic floor to the top of the head, following the line of points of energy.

SAT NAM – Used in Kundalini yoga, this mantra opens the door to intuition, reinvigorates sexual energy, and awakens the body's chakra energy points. To say it properly, the SAT is drawn out in length to be eight times longer than the NAM.

OM SHANTI – This mantra is said to be the sound of the universe and cosmic vibration. The word "Shanti" comes from the Sanskrit "peace," "calm," or "bliss."

SO-HUM – This mantra follows the pattern of the breath by matching the vibration of the inhale and the exhale to create a sense of calm awareness.

I AM – This is a great mantra for morning meditation.

OM MANI PADME HUM – This is a longer mantra that means, "The jewel is in the lotus." It may also mean, "Praise the jewel in the lotus." It is said slowly.

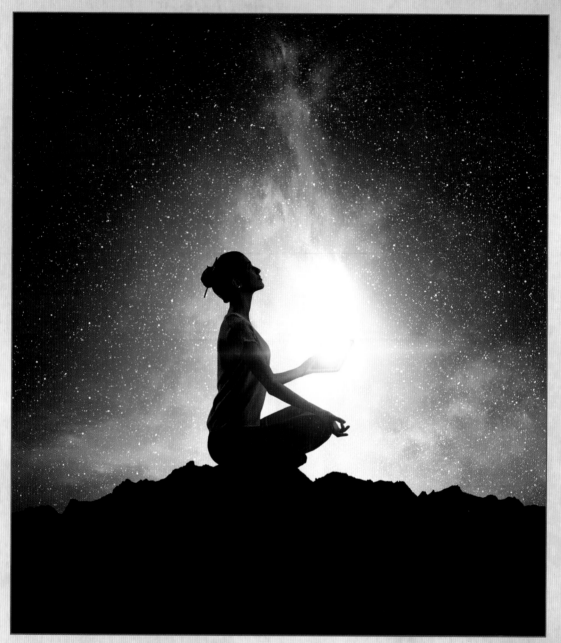

Any word or words can be a mantra, but they must mean something to you, be repeated deliberately, and keep your mind from wandering. Those who like a visual aid rather than words can meditate with eyes open and focused upon the burning flame of a candle, a beautiful piece of art, a symbolic and sacred object, or a waterfall or natural setting. Again, the idea is to stay focused on the visual aid, free from distractions.

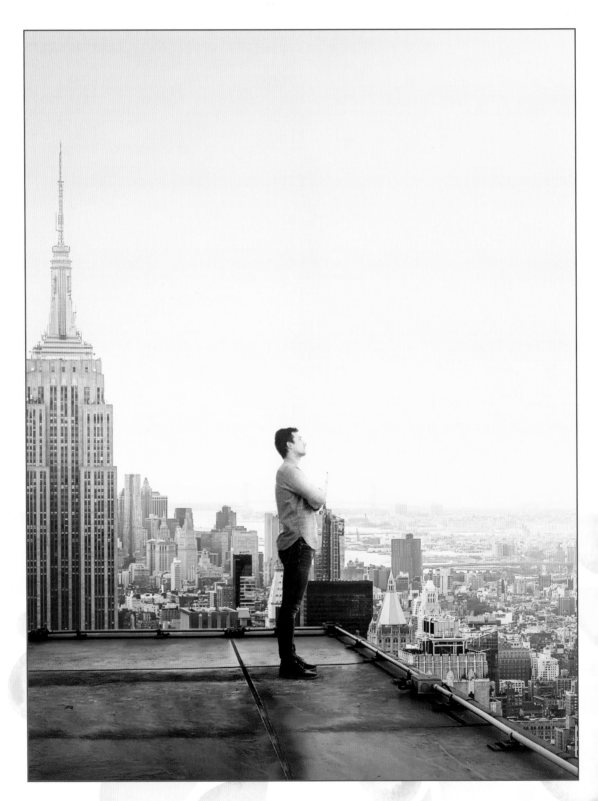

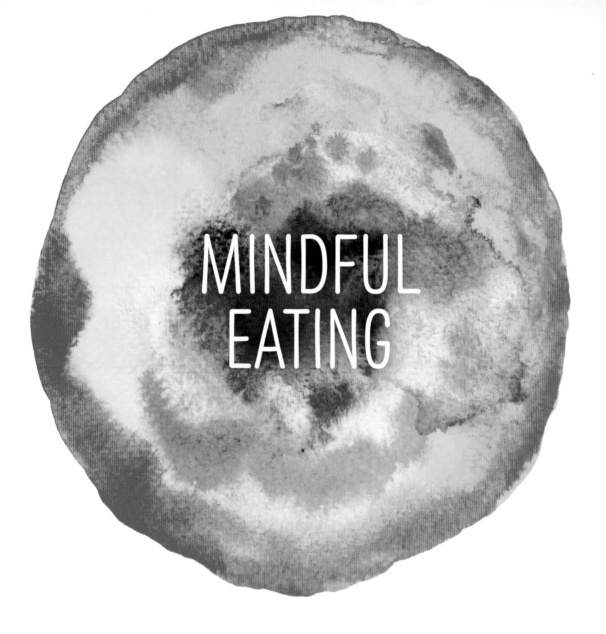

# MINDFUL EATING

In the early 20th century, a self-proclaimed nutritionist and businessman by the name of Horace Fletcher proposed some interesting ideas about eating. Fletcher believed that during a meal, each bite of food should be thoroughly chewed—approximately 32 chews per bite, one bite for each tooth—before being swallowed. He even suggested that the same chewing effort should be given to liquids, so beverages would be pre-mixed with saliva before they were swallowed. All of this chewing, he believed, would help to jump-start the digestion process and help the body absorb nutrients without absorbing as many calories. Fletcher also told his followers that they should eat only when hungry, and they should refrain from eating when feeling angry or sad. And, he said, they should pay attention to what sorts of ingredients were in their food, as different foods produced different "waste products."

Fletcher was nicknamed "The Great Masticator" by his followers, and the practice of chewing food to the point of near-obliteration was coined "Fletcherizing." Adherents made sure to Fletcherize at every meal, believing it to be best for their health and digestive systems. Eventually, Fletcher's unusual concepts were replaced with the still-popular notion of counting calories. But even today, the father of Fletcherizing is attached to the catchy tagline: "Nature will castigate those who don't masticate."

Chewing a bite of food dozens of times does seem like a bit of overkill. But it turns out that Fletcher may have been on to something. Surprisingly, studies have found that when people chew their food more, they end up eating up to 12 percent fewer calories overall. And it's hard to argue with the logic of only eating when hungry, or of being aware of what sorts

of ingredients are in the foods we put into our bodies. These ideas may have seemed "radical" in the Victorian era, but nowadays they line right up with what nutritionists and dietitians preach. Fletcher was even on the right track when he advocated abstaining from eating when feeling emotional. In fact, the struggle of emotional eating has led to its own niche within the $20 billion weight loss industry, and gyms and weight loss clinics are full of people struggling not to feed their emotions and overeat.

In a way, Horace Fletcher may have been ahead of his time. While The Great Masticator is mostly remembered as the creator of a fad diet, it's not far off to say that he was also, perhaps inadvertently, one of the first practitioners of mindful eating.

## FAST-PACED FIASCO

If you're like many people, chances are you don't always eat in a mindful way. Think about a typical day with typical mealtimes. Breakfast might be rushed as you hurry to get yourself and the rest of your household out the door. Maybe you grab a quick slice of toast or a bowl of cereal, or just down a glass of juice before heading out. Or perhaps you eat something in your car during your commute, while

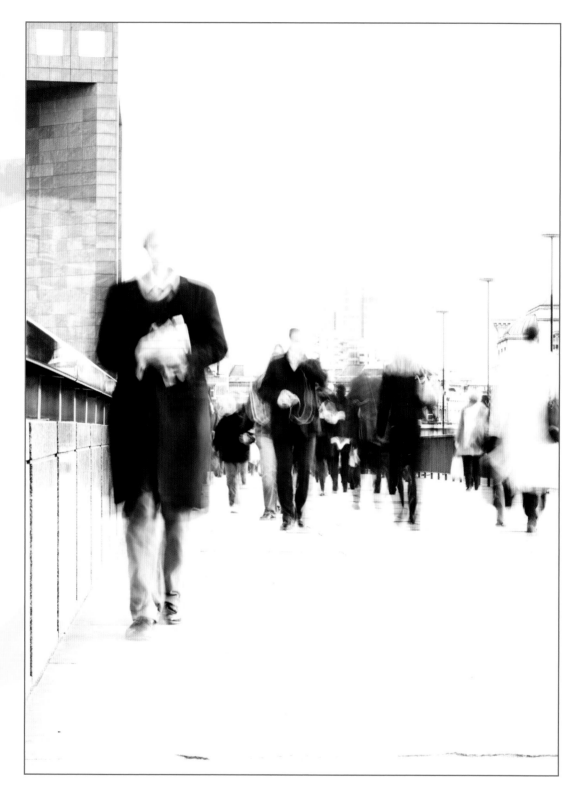

you attempt not to dribble jam on your outfit or leave crumbs on the console. You probably swig some coffee, not really paying much attention to it. You just hope the caffeine rush will hit and give you energy to get through the rest of the morning.

Lunch may be at your desk at work, where you don't necessarily take a real break. You continue to read emails or peruse reports or take phone calls, your lunch scattered over your desk. You absentmindedly take bites of a sandwich, or maybe reach into a bag of chips, chomping through them until all you're left with is crumbs. Except by the time you finish, you hardly remember eating the whole bag—where did all those chips go? When afternoon rolls around, you feel sluggish and tired and in need of a pick-me-up. So you grab another cup of coffee, or hit up the vending machine and buy a bag of cookies or some candy. And once again you eat your snack at your desk, where work is occupying most of your attention and the snack is just an afterthought. When it disappears, you hardly remember where it went.

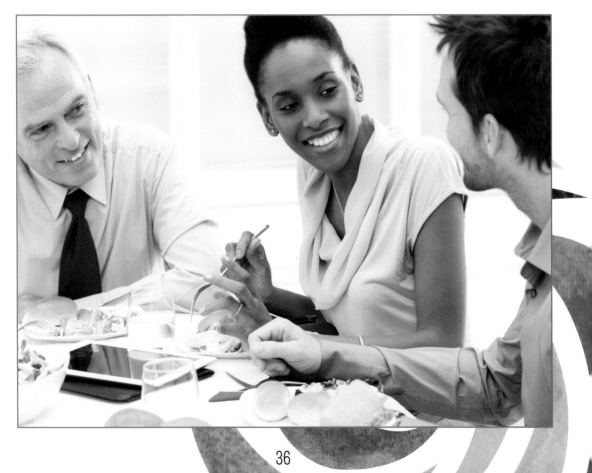

By the time you're home and ready for dinner, you're tired and hungry. Maybe you don't even feel like cooking, so you just throw something in the microwave. Or perhaps you order out and have food delivered. Either way, you end up in front of the television, a plate on your lap, watching your favorite show and paying more attention to the screen than whatever you're putting in your mouth. You wind up with empty dishes, but not much recollection of how your meal tasted. And then there's the late night snack—you probably don't even need another handful of chips or a bowl of ice cream, but perhaps it's just become habit to grab something to eat while you watch evening talk shows and unwind.

Many of us eat our meals in this way. We try to be great multitaskers, so we combine mealtimes with other errands and responsibilities, like driving or reading emails or folding laundry. Even when we eat foods that we might perceive as a "reward"— like a decadent brownie after a tough day at the office, or a cheeseburger at a summer cookout—we can be left feeling weirdly unsatisfied when our treat is finished.

Even worse is when we "indulge" in some kind of "diet" food—food that

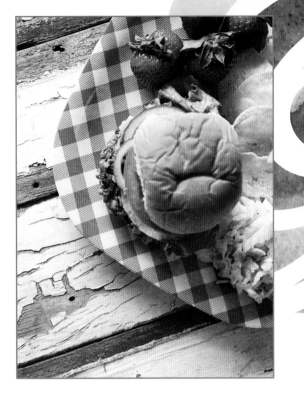

has been made "better" or lower calorie by replacing fat and sugar with artificial ingredients. Have you ever noticed that a "low-fat, low-sugar" cookie is nowhere near as satisfying as the real deal? And when one of those diet cookies doesn't bring us the same kind of satisfaction we get from its higher-calorie counterparts, we might eat a few more just to see if quantity can trump quality.

The result of all this mindless eating is, at best, a lack of appreciation for the abundant food we are fortunate to have. But at worst, it can lead to weight gain and a sense of dissatisfaction with mealtimes.

And if you're not satisfied after you eat, what tends to happen? More eating. Which leads to more weight gain. The cycle is obvious, but as all those gym goers and weight loss center members can attest to, it can be difficult to break the cycle. That's where mindful eating can step in. So what exactly is mindful eating? And how can it help us develop a healthier relationship to our food?

## A SINGLE RAISIN

Many of the principles behind mindful eating are similar to those we use for general mindfulness. When we practice mindfulness, we try to use all of our senses to observe the present moment. With

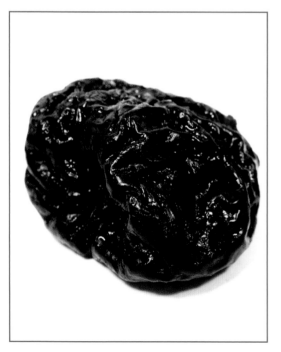

mindful eating, we do the same. Instead of eating food without thought to what we're doing, we deliberately pay attention to each bite, taking note of the appearance, smell, texture, taste, and even sound of the food we eat. And just as we approach our emotions in a non-judgmental way when we practice mindfulness, we do the same with mindful eating—we try not to think of any particular food as "good" or "bad," and we taste foods without allowing our perception of them to alter our experience.

In their book, *The Mindful Way through Depression: Freeing Yourself from Chronic Unhappiness*, authors Mark Williams, John Teasdale, Zindel Segal, and Jon Kabat-Zinn use the example of eating one single raisin to describe the nuances of mindful eating. Through an eight-step process, they describe how we can practice mindful eating even with the tiniest bites of food. So grab a raisin—or, if you don't have any raisins in your pantry, feel free to use a grape, a single corn flake, a chocolate chip, or any other small bite of food—and try out a quick mindful eating exercise.

The first step is to simply hold the food item. Place it between your thumb and finger as you move on to step two: see it.

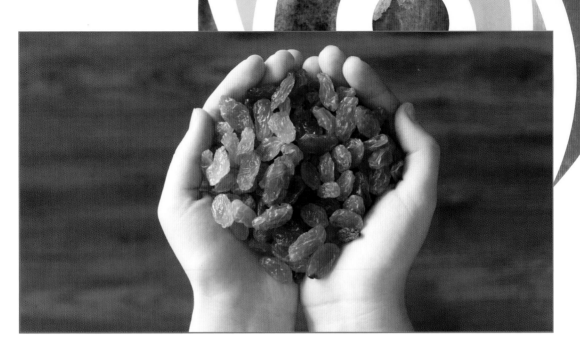

Look at the raisin and pay attention to what you see. Take note of the curves and ridges of the fruit. Now spend a few moments observing the texture—turn the raisin over in your fingers, using your sense of touch. Next, engage your sense of smell: Hold the raisin to your nose, and inhale the fragrance. What does it smell like?

Now it's time to place the raisin in your mouth—but don't chew it. Just observe the sensation of the food in your mouth and the way it feels on your tongue. Next, begin to chew slowly, taking note of where the raisin is in your mouth, and what the first taste is like. Notice how the texture changes as you chew. When you feel like you're ready, swallow the raisin. And finally, follow

up the whole exercise by observing anything you feel afterwards. Can you feel the raisin as it travels down your esophagus? How has eating a single raisin in this mindful way made you feel?

Eating mindfully in this way can help us to enjoy our food more, which can actually help us to feel satisfied even when we eat less. With our hectic lifestyles, we have a tendency to want to accomplish as much as possible in as short a time as possible. When it comes to eating, we see it almost as an afterthought—something we can do anytime, anywhere. But when we eat without paying attention, it can have unintended consequences. After all, eating is a more complicated endeavor than it

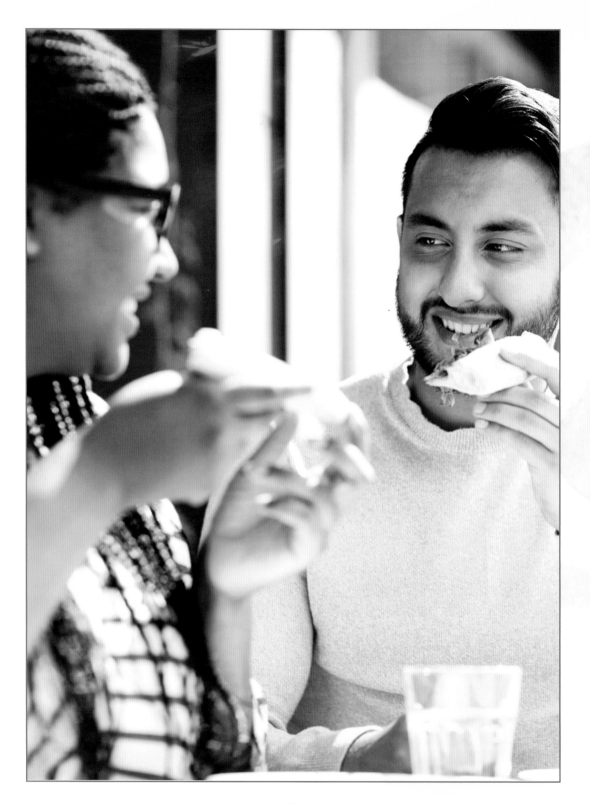

appears. If it were a simple case of providing our bodies with fuel, the issues of obesity and overeating wouldn't be as likely to arise.

One of the things that makes eating more complicated is the hormone that regulates fullness. The intestinal tract secretes a hormone called ghrelin to signal your brain that it's time to stop eating. The problem? Experts have noted that it takes about 20 minutes for the ghrelin signal to reach the brain and cause you to feel "full." So when we eat quickly, or without paying attention, we risk overeating before we even realize we're full. We end up with that uncomfortable bloated feeling, and probably a mind full of regret.

Not only that, but when we eat mindlessly, our food is much less enjoyable. If we're eating a sweet layer cake or a succulent steak dinner, why would we want to distract ourselves with work or television programs? Wouldn't we rather savor each bite?

Our modern lifestyle doesn't help the matter. Food is everywhere! Decades ago, it took much more time and effort to acquire groceries, and people ate foods that they prepared themselves. Nowadays, we can buy food at the corner grocery store, in drugstores, at coffee shops, or even when we're filling up the

car with gas—and it's usually pre-packaged convenience food that is ready to eat. We don't have to go any farther than back to the car to start eating, which we do while we're driving to our next destination, listening to the radio, and fighting traffic.

Mindful eating can help us not only fuel our bodies with the nutrients it needs, but also enjoy the experience. So what are some of the principles behind mindful eating?

## SLOW DOWN

One of the most basic ideas—and perhaps most important—is to slow down. Many times we eat quickly, without even thinking about it. And even when we finally get a chance to relax, we may not realize at times how quickly we eat. We sit down in front of the television with a bag of chips, and before we've even finished watching a show, the bag is empty. Mindful eating requires a slower pace—you need time to pay attention to what you're eating, so you can engage your senses and savor the experience.

You may not always have the time to devote to mindful eating, and that's OK. Sometimes mornings are rushed and work is busy, and it's not always practical to sit down and eat slowly. But try to set aside at least one or two meals a week for mindful eating, and you may find that you enjoy it so much that you strive to do it more often.

## LOSE THE DISTRACTIONS

You should also try to eat without distractions. In other words, don't multitask while you're eating. Try not to eat in the car. Step away from the computer during lunch. Turn off the television before dinner. You can also put your phone on silent, or leave it in another room so you're not tempted to scroll through social media while you eat. This makes it easier to pay attention—not only to what your food smells and tastes like, but to how you feel as you're

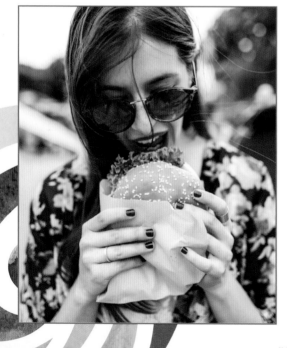

eating. You'll be better able to recognize when you're full if you're not distracted by work or noise.

## PAY ATTENTION TO HUNGER CUES

Another principle of mindful eating is using hunger cues to dictate when you should eat. This may seem obvious, but how often do we actually pay attention to whether or not we're actually hungry? Eating when we're not hungry seems to be another byproduct of our convenient society—since food is constantly available, we don't think twice about eating, whether or not we want or need to. Think about that box of cookies in the office break room, or the snacks you keep in the pantry "for the kids." How many times have you walked past an abundance of snack food and grabbed some without even thinking about it? If you're like many of us, it happens more often than you'd like to admit.

This is not to say that you shouldn't eat until you're starving—this can be its own danger, because ravenous hunger can lead to crankiness and poor decisions. Instead of making a healthy choice to eat, you're more likely to reach for some convenient junk food and devour it before you have time to consider whether it's

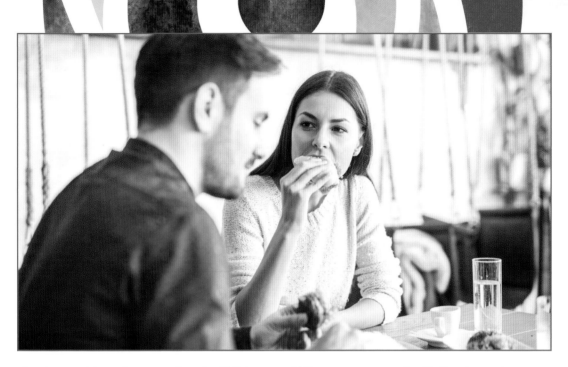

the best thing for your body. With mindful eating, the key is to pay close attention to your own body's hunger cues. Mindfulness teaches us to pause before we act—this is a useful lesson to embrace with mindful eating. Pause before you reach for a snack, and ask yourself whether you really need it. Sometimes the answer will be yes, and that's OK—but many times, you'll discover that your desire for food is simply stemming from boredom or stress.

## DON'T JUDGE

Mindfulness teaches us that there are no "bad" or "good" feelings. So it's not surprising that the same idea applies to mindful eating.

When we eat mindfully, there is no such thing as "good" food or "bad" food. Rather, with mindful eating, we attempt to recognize the foods that will nourish us, while also appreciating the foods that simply taste good. When all food is given an even plane, none of it seems "forbidden" or more "virtuous" than any other. It becomes easier to eat a healthy diet, while also realizing that treats and special indulgences aren't off-limits. In fact, in our attempt to make foods that we've deemed "bad" into "good" foods, we've really sabotaged ourselves. Supermarket aisles are lined with "low-fat" cookies and ice cream, the results of our desire to be "better" about what we eat. But if you had the choice between two or three low-fat cookies made with a few

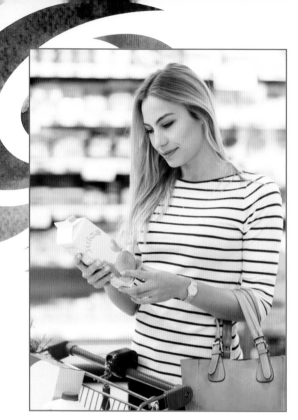

bite of food and decide you "hate" it, you accept your reaction without judgment. Likewise, when you "love" a food, you simply acknowledge the feeling and move on.

## USE YOUR SENSES

Lastly, when we eat mindfully, we use all of our senses. Think back to the single raisin example: You not only tasted the raisin, but you looked at it, touched it, and smelled it, as well. You can even engage your sense of hearing with some foods—crunchy carrots, for example, or the light crack of the caramelized sugar on a crème brûlée—the point is to just pay attention to the entire experience when you eat, instead of mindlessly putting food in your mouth. You may discover that there is so much more to enjoy about eating than simply the taste of food.

unpronounceable ingredients or one regular cookie made with butter and chocolate and vanilla, which would you chose? Chances are, you'd want one single regular cookie, because even the ingredients sound delicious, and it would be much more satisfying. So when we buy those low-fat cookies, with the intention to eat "better," we may end up eating even more than we would if we simply stuck to regular cookies, because one of the "better" cookies isn't nearly as satisfying.

And once again, just as with mindfulness, we practice non-judgment when eating mindfully. This means that when you take a

So now that you know some of the principles of the practice, how can mindful eating be helpful? Let's start by exploring the first principle—slowing down.

Years ago, in the late 1980s, researchers noticed something interesting about the people of France. Even though the French diet was high in foods like cheese, butter, and pastries, French people had a lower risk of obesity. Even today, obesity rates in France are about half of what they are in the United States. Yet French croissants are famous for their copious amounts of butter; French wine is coveted by many a sommelier. How can the French eat cheese and croissants and not struggle with the obesity rates of the U.S.?

Part of the answer may lie in how the French approach mealtimes. If you were to visit a French restaurant for lunch, scarf down your meal quickly, and then impatiently signal the waiter for your bill, you might be perceived as a rude patron. This is because in France, a lunch at a restaurant can stretch on for two hours. People take the time to enjoy

their food, by savoring one bite at a time before moving on to another. Eating this way can actually make our food taste better, as well. Have you ever noticed that your first bite of chocolate cake tastes much better than the last? This is because our taste buds "tire out" after tasting the same thing over and over.

Another way the French get it right is by serving smaller portions. Sure, they eat cheese and pastries, but they eat less of them. And remember, it takes about 20 minutes for your body to tell your brain that you're full. By slowing down and focusing on each bite, and taking the time your body needs to process the meal, it takes less food to feel more satisfied. You can eat a smaller portion and still feel like you had plenty to eat.

As we've talked about, it's important to rid yourself of distractions when practicing mindful eating. And researchers are discovering that eating without distractions may be even more important than anyone realized. The things we do throughout the day are stored in our mind's memory bank—we can think back over whatever happened during the day, and those memories shape our reactions and thoughts and feelings. When we eat in a distracted manner, our brains may only record the other things we are doing—driving, or replying to emails, for instance—and we "forget" that we ate anything at all. Once again, we eat an entire meal, but we end up feeling unsatisfied because the experience hasn't been stored in our memory. Even more troubling, there is evidence that eating while distracted actually slows the digestion process. We're left with another negative cycle: We eat while we're distracted, which leaves us unsatisfied. So we eat more, even though our digestive system is still working on our previous meal!

Our eating habits aren't all that suffer when we eat distractedly—we're less effective at our jobs when we attempt to eat and work at the same time, too. So don't feel guilty for taking that entire lunch hour—you'll be satisfied with your meal, and you'll be more productive when you get back to work!

## EMOTIONAL EATING

Now let's talk about another principle of mindful eating: paying attention to hunger cues.
This isn't always as simple as "I'm hungry" or "I'm not hungry." As we already mentioned, the act of eating is more complicated than it seems like it should be. Horace Fletcher was certainly on to something when he told his followers

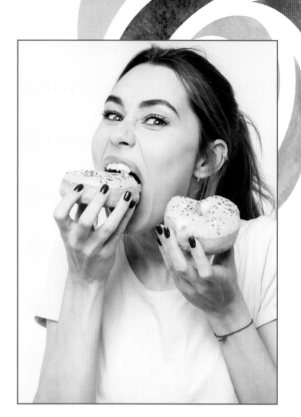

that they should refrain from eating during moments of anger or sadness. Emotional eating is a genuine problem. Who hasn't turned to food during times of stress? We feel upset about something, so we head to the freezer and pull out a pint of ice cream, maybe digging our spoon straight into the carton. Perhaps we're exhausted from a long day, and the thought of cooking is too much; we randomly snack on whatever catches our eye until we've rummaged through half the pantry. Or maybe we're just feeling bored, and that leftover cake seems to be calling to us from its stand on the counter.

All of these are examples of emotional eating, and chances are, you've run into one (or all) of these situations at one time or another. And while it's not always a bad thing to simply eat for the sake of eating—perhaps at a party or special occasion—when it becomes a habit, it can be a problem. You begin to associate your feelings with food, and eating for emotional reasons creates an unhealthy cycle. Emotional hunger and physical hunger are not the same thing, and mindful eating can help you sort through the differences.

## BATTLING EMOTIONAL EATING

Food does more than provide energy and fill us up. It is also a source of how we often deal with our feelings. It may be a bowl of ice cream when we're happy, a box of cookies when we're sad, or a bag of chips when we're just bored. But when we eat even though we aren't hungry, we're engaging in emotional eating. The reason we do it is because eating causes our bodies to release dopamine to our brain's reward centers. This helps us feel less sad or get more pleasure when we're happy. But it can be an easy trap to fall into when we're trying to lose weight.

The best way to steer clear of emotional eating is to learn how to recognize its telltale signs. Emotional

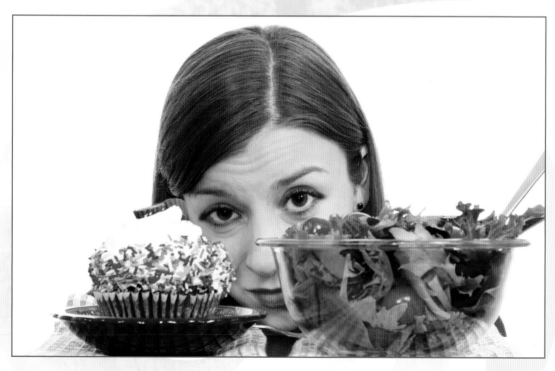

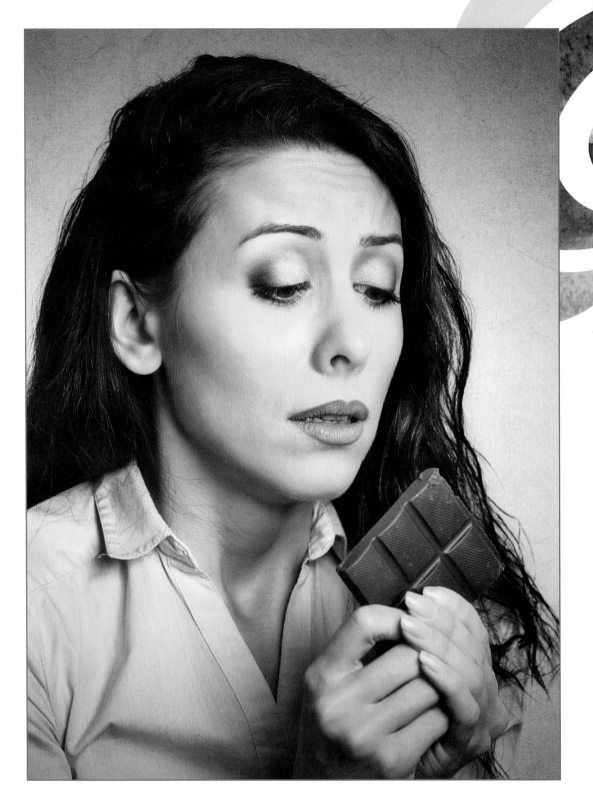

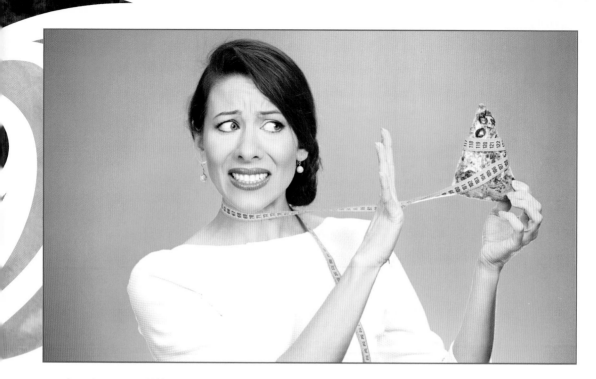

eating is very different than eating because of physical hunger. You can easily identify it for what it is. Emotional hunger happens very suddenly, while physical hunger builds up gradually. Emotional hunger also feels like you need to satisfy it as soon as possible. Physical hunger can be ignored at least for a short while. If you find yourself craving a specific comfort food, like ice cream or chips, and only that food is going to satisfy you, then you're probably eating emotionally. When you are eating because of physical hunger, you are willing to consider several options. And even when you feel full, if you're eating emotionally, you want to continue eating. Finally, emotional eating often leaves you feeling guilty, while eating to satisfy physical hunger doesn't.

When you are tempted to engage in emotional eating, identify the emotion that you're experiencing and identify the circumstances that caused it. Then, put your plan into action. Remind yourself of your short-term and long-term goals. Write down your feelings in a journal. And take steps to alleviate the emotions you're experiencing without using comfort food.

Combating stress is an important part of preventing emotional eating. Stress in one form or another is often the trigger for emotional eating, whether we're aware of a particular set of circumstances that led to

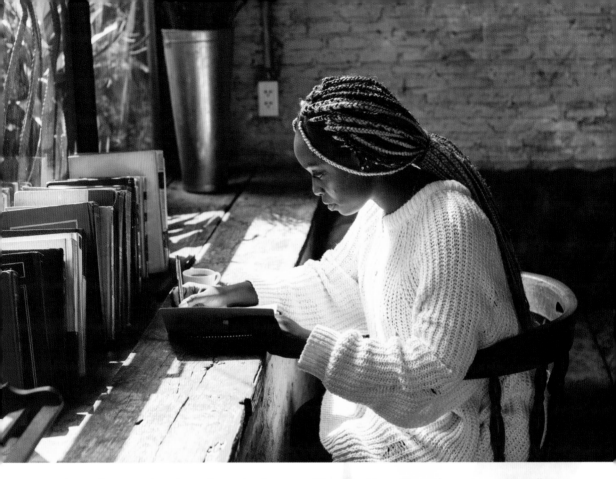

such eating or simply exhausted after a day full of low-level but constant stress. Fortunately, there are a few things you can do to reduce the amount of stress you're experiencing.

**Get more sleep.** A lack of sleep will not only leave you without the energy you need to make it through your day, it can make you stressed out. When you aren't getting enough sleep, your body is producing more cortisol. And if you're stressed out all day, you'll actually have more trouble getting a good night's rest, leading to a self-perpetuating cycle.

**Stay active.** Regular exercise will help lower the levels of cortisol in your bloodstream. Exercise also causes your brain to release endorphins and dopamine. This is the reason for the "runner's high," and it can work for you, too—and you don't need to run a marathon to experience its benefits. You'll notice that you feel better and more centered immediately after you exercise and for some time after, even if you exercise for as little as ten minutes. Chapter four explores mindfulness and exercise in some more detail.

You should also identify sources of stress and avoid them whenever possible. If you can't avoid them altogether, develop strategies to prevent them from ruining your day. Maybe it's the gridlock or the packed subway car on your way to work. Maybe it's someone at your work. Or it could be any number of other triggers. Identify the ones you can cut out of your life, and you'll be better equipped to deal with the ones you can't.

## ASSEMBLING A TOOLKIT

Anyone who has ever tried to change their eating habits knows all too well that it's really tough to do without a plan, clear goals, and a lot of support. Changing your lifestyle is not something that can be done overnight, and it's not something that can be done by yourself. Even with the best of intentions and a lot of motivation, if you don't prepare resources and strategies that can keep you going, it will be very difficult to succeed. That's why it's important to assemble a set of tools you can use to develop your new lifestyle and maintain it over the long term. So before we move on, let's put your toolkit together.

One of the most important things that should be in your toolkit is a positive attitude. Remember, this lifestyle is not one of those deprivation diets that revolve around negative body image, guilt, or self-shaming—so start getting rid of those right now! Instead, fill your toolkit with positive thinking, self-love, and respect for your body. Make sure to revisit these positive thoughts on a daily basis so that you are regularly reminding yourself of what you have chosen to do. The positive thinking that you keep in your toolkit should focus on what you love about your body. Think about how your body helps you accomplish goals and finish tasks as you go through your day. Remember that your body is beautiful. And keep in mind that you're taking control of your lifestyle and empowering yourself to make food choices and develop habits that will help you live a longer, healthier, and happier life.

The next addition to your toolkit is a set of strategies to deal with stress when it does occur. The first strategy, as mentioned already, is simply to sleep more. If you regularly skimp on sleep, you're going to be stressed before you even make it out the door in the morning. Sleep is essential to being able to keep your stress levels low. The good news is that once you get on a regular sleep schedule, your body will quickly adjust, and getting enough sleep will become second nature. We'll talk more about sleep in chapter seven.

Second, try to determine what things cause you the most stress on a daily basis, and develop ways to minimize your exposure to them. If you can identify the stressors that irk you regularly, you'll be able to plan strategies to either avoid them altogether, or if that isn't possible, distance yourself from them.

Third, find allies you can rely on to help you recharge your batteries when you've had a stressful day. Wherever you can, surround yourself with people whose company leaves you feeling happy and relaxed, and avoid people who leave you emotionally drained after you spend time with them. Your friends and/or significant other should be people you're able to lean on for emotional support, reaffirmation, and comfort.

Having people you can rely on in your circle is crucial for both combating stress and helping you succeed in your new lifestyle. When you're embarking on a healthy lifestyle change and developing better habits, having the support of those around you is critical. The worst thing you can do is not tell anyone that you're trying to eat better and get more exercise. You should share your goals and reasons for your

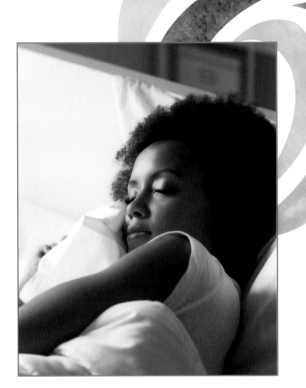

new lifestyle with the people you care about; you'll be pleasantly surprised by how eager they'll be to give you support.

Trust your friends and family to be supportive, and give them the tools they need to help you succeed. Feel free to have heartfelt conversations with them about why you're doing this and ask them for specific ways they can help you. You may need to avoid certain restaurants your family is used to frequenting or keep trigger foods out of the house for a while. Or you may have to tell your friends that you'd rather get together for activities that involve taking walks or bike rides together, rather than going to happy hour at the bar.

The final piece of your toolkit is your calendar. More specifically, it's time cleared on your calendar for exercise. Maintaining an exercise program is only possible if you make time for it. That means drawing a big, red circle around the time of day you plan on doing your exercises and not letting anything else inside of it. Turn the phone off, make sure your friends and family know that that 30 or 45 minutes of the day is yours alone, and tell them (kindly) that you simply aren't available then.

In order to make sure your exercise schedule is sustainable, you have to clear time for it in advance. Instead of trying to carve out time for exercise on a day-to-day basis, plan ahead, set a schedule, and do your best to stick to it (but don't be hard on yourself if you slip up—remember, nobody's perfect). Have a number of exercise routines that you can fit easily into busy schedules. Find out what time of day you feel most comfortable exercising. Whatever time works for you is fine—just make sure it's a time that you can consistently stick with. See chapter four for a variety of exercise ideas.

Are you feeling motivated? Start looking forward to the changes you're going to introduce to your lifestyle. It's going to be amazing!

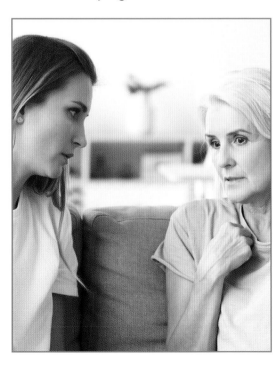

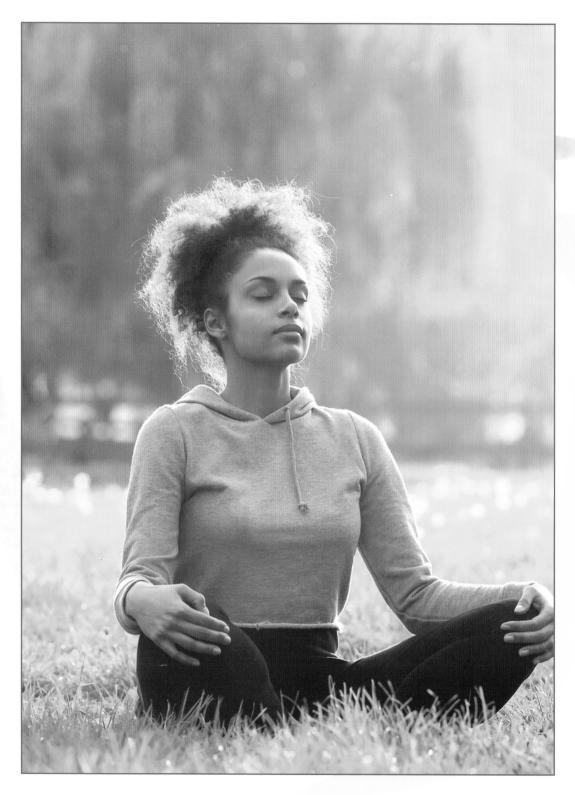

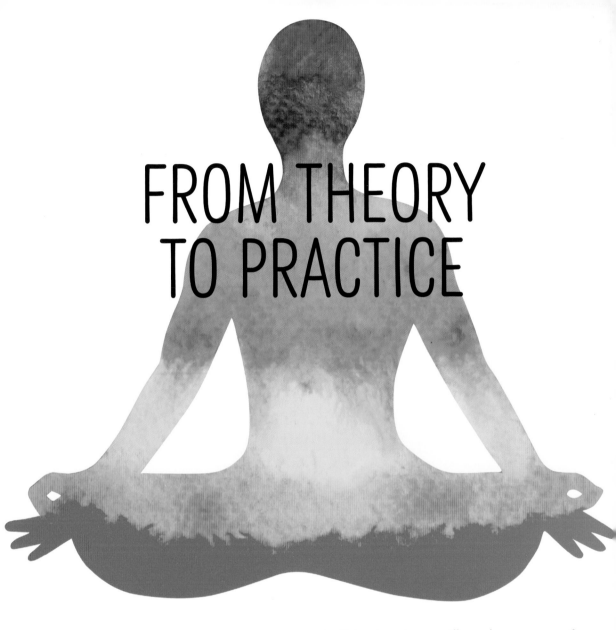

# FROM THEORY TO PRACTICE

## MINDFUL EATING, MINDFUL LIVING

As you practice mindful eating, you can focus on making sure you're bringing excellent nutritious food to your body.

In this chapter, we'll explore some of those foods that will make you feel great, stay healthy, and maintain energy throughout the day. The foods highlighted in this section are not only superb additions to your diet, but they are also excellent starting points for a more mindful existence.

We'll conclude the section with six scrumptious recipes that make use of many of the following foods.

**Oils** are one such starting point. Recommended oils include canola, safflower, sesame, soybean, flaxseed, sunflower, olive, and peanut. Flaxseed oil is an excellent source of an acid that your body converts into omega-3 fatty acids. Olive oil not only has all of the health benefits found in the Mediterranean diet studies, but it is also a powerful antibacterial agent that can help keep your stomach biota balanced and healthy. Olive oil also contains oleocanthol, a compound that has similar properties to those found in nonsteroidal anti-inflammatory drugs such as Ibuprofen, which may be the reason it is associated with lower rates of heart disease.

The oil you choose for each meal will be based on what you're using it for. If you're cooking, you'll want to use oil that has a smoke point at or near the temperature you will be cooking at. Unrefined oils have lower smoke points than refined oils; soybean and safflower oils have some of the highest smoke points. If you're drizzling the oil over your meal, you'll want to choose based on flavor.

**Olives** are extraordinarily versatile. There are dozens of varieties of olives from around the world.

You can find an olive variety to complement almost any meal. Olives can be stuffed, added to salads, made into dips and spreads, or simply enjoyed as a light snack. Olives, rich in monounsaturated fats, are also an excellent source of vitamin E, iron, and other minerals. They contain antioxidants, anti-inflammatory compounds, and hydroxytyrosol, a nutrient that is associated with cancer prevention.

**Nuts and seeds** are perhaps the broadest category of healthy monounsaturated fatty acid (MUFA)-rich foods. The nutritional benefits of seeds and nuts are myriad. Walnuts are high in omega-3 fatty acids and contain the highest levels of antioxidants of any nut, and they contain manganese, which may help reduce premenstrual symptoms. Almonds have more fiber than other nuts and are extremely rich in vitamin E, another great antioxidant. Almonds have also been shown to help with weight loss, in part because they're rich in MUFAs, but also due to their high fiber content.

Cashews are rich in zinc and iron, and can help boost brain function. An ounce of cashews also provides 25% of your daily recommendation of magnesium, which has been shown to help memory function. Brazil nuts are rich in selenium, which can help prevent certain cancers.

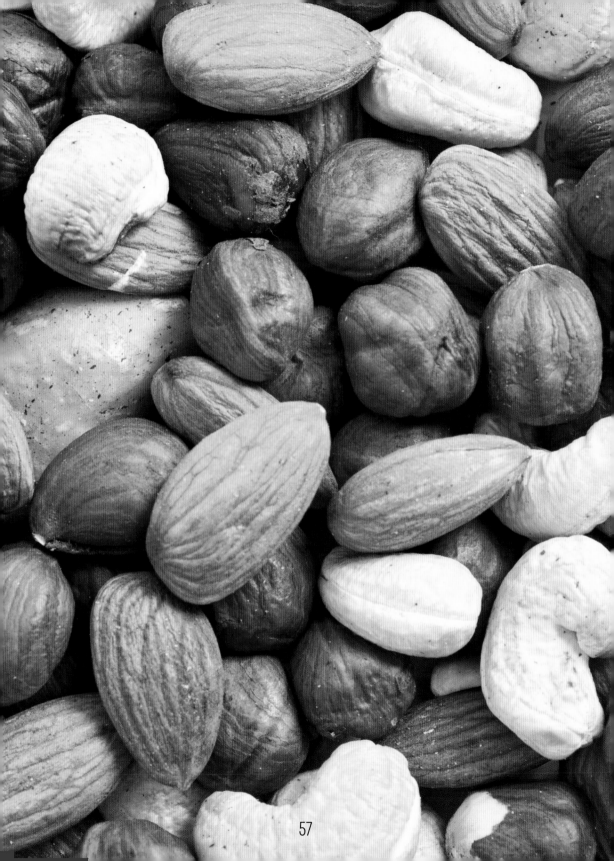

Macadamia nuts have the highest MUFA content. Pistachios help you burn calories while you eat them—they don't come out of their shell willingly, which helps you slow down consumption and eat less overall. They are also rich in cancer-fighting antioxidants, and contain a lot of vitamin B6, which can help boost your mood and strengthen your immune system.

Pumpkin seeds are a tasty source of vitamin B and minerals such as magnesium, iron, and zinc. They also contain an amino acid called tryptophan, which can help reduce anxiety. And they're packed with monounsaturated fats. Sunflower seeds provide an excellent source

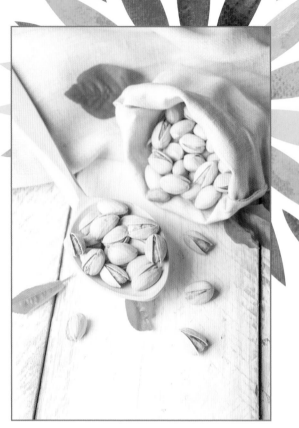

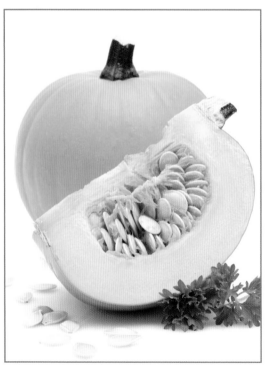

of several B vitamins, including folate, which is critical to healthy pregnancy and boosts the immune system. They're also rich in vitamin E, and can help maintain healthy skin and hair and may prevent certain cancers. Flax seeds are chock-full of nutritional benefits; they are simply bursting with omega-3 fatty acids, help stabilize blood sugar, and contain lignans, which may be linked to preventing cancer.

The best thing about nuts and seeds is their amazing versatility in the kitchen. You can sprinkle them over salads or toast them to add rich flavor to just about any meal. You can add nuts to yogurt or smoothies to add texture and flavor, or simply pack some as trail mix to help you get through the day.

**Avocados** are practically a perfect food. They are packed with potassium, vitamins A and E, and monounsaturated fat. They also contain some vitamin B and C along with a little protein and starch. They are rich in fiber and vitamin K, which is critical to blood clotting, potassium, and folate. Avocados are an excellent source of antioxidants (excellent for heart and cardiovascular health), and contain anti-aging properties as well. They

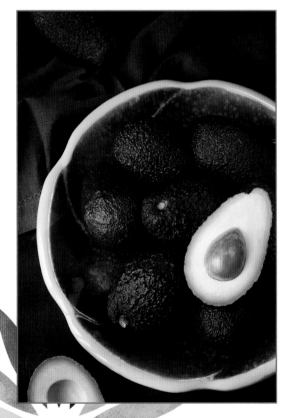

also have been shown to help the body to absorb carotenoids, an antioxidant found in other vegetables that lowers the risk of heart disease. Avocados are also rich in lutein, which has been linked to optical health.

You can eat an avocado all by itself for a quick, satisfying snack, or incorporate it into a full meal. You can make a delicious guacamole to enjoy with friends or spread on a sandwich, or slice an avocado to complement a salad or serve as a side to breakfast, lunch, or dinner. When you are picking out an avocado at the grocery store, try to find one that gives ever so slightly when you squeeze it.

**Dark chocolate** is a perfect accompaniment to a healthy lifestyle; not only is it rich in monounsaturated fats, it's got a full complement of additional nutrients as well. It's an excellent source of HDL-boosting molecules like flavanols. It also helps your body regulate insulin levels, lowers your blood pressure, and is loaded with minerals such as copper, magnesium, potassium, calcium, and iron.

Dark chocolate has a much lower sugar content than other chocolate. It isn't as sweet as other kinds of chocolate, but it has a rich, pungent

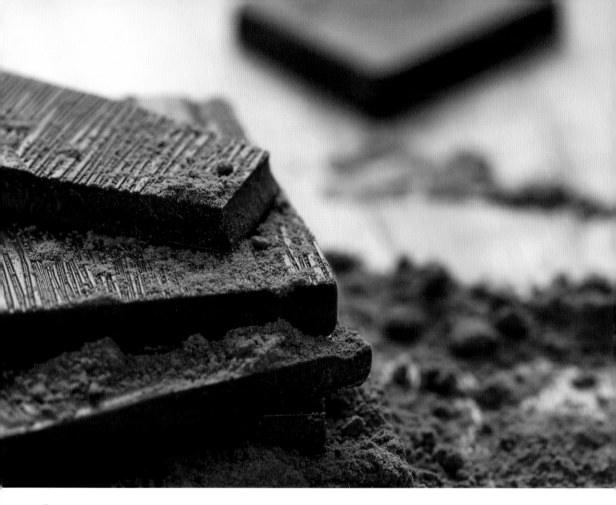

flavor that has to be experienced to be appreciated. If you've never tried dark chocolate, you're in for a treat—but don't start yourself off with the darkest chocolate you can find. Gradually acquire a taste for dark chocolate by starting off with something that is about 60 percent cacao, and gradually work your way up to the stronger stuff. After a while, you may even prefer dark chocolate to anything else.

## OTHER FOODS

Make an effort to get one of the foods listed above into each meal or snack you eat. But what about other foods? Here are some other powerhouse food choices.

**Blueberries** were a staple for Native Americans, who introduced them to European settlers. Blueberries are a delicious source of vitamin C, and they're also one of the best sources of antioxidants as well. They have higher amounts of antioxidant chemicals than red wine. They have been shown to help memory function and may even help prevent Alzheimer's and other forms of dementia. They're also great for circulation and heart health, help relieve stress, and can aid digestion. Fresh blueberries are a yummy addition to smoothies or breakfast cereal, and they're great to pack for a midday snack to help raise blood sugar levels, boost energy and mood, and fend off cravings. Try to only purchase organic blueberries, and if you can't get them, wash your berries before you eat them.

**Eggs** have long been considered bad in light of their high cholesterol content, but the truth is they don't actually contribute to elevated levels of total or LDL cholesterol in the bloodstream. Eggs are backed with nutrients and come pre-packaged for easy portability. They contain zinc and iron, which can strengthen nails and hair, and have carotenoids that have been shown to help reduce macular degeneration, which is a major cause of vision loss among elderly adults. Eggs are rich in lecithin, which in turn contains choline. Choline helps move cholesterol through the bloodstream, helping to prevent plaque from developing. Egg yolks are one of the few sources of vitamin D, which can help reduce

the risk of heart disease and certain forms of cancer, boost immune function, and prevent diabetes. Eggs also provide vitamins A, B, and B12 in particular. And eggs are a "complete protein," that is, they contain all nine of the essential amino acids that your body does not produce.
Eggs can complement any meal or serve as a snack all on their own. Whether scrambled, poached, or cooked into an omelet, eggs make a great breakfast. Or you can hard boil an egg and pack it for a quick snack in the middle of the day. When you're buying eggs, look for free-range labels. Free-range eggs have slightly higher levels of carotenoids and are often a bit bigger and have richer yolks as well.

**Whole grains** are an excellent source of nutrients. Unlike white flour, which has the bran and germ removed from the grain, whole grain flour is ground from grains that retain the bran and germ. Depending on what kind of grain it is, between 50 and 90 percent of the nutrients and phytochemicals in the plant are contained in the bran and germ. Each part of the plant contributes different nutrients, so it's much better for your long-term health, disease prevention, and overall digestion to eat whole grains. People who eat at least three servings of whole grains each

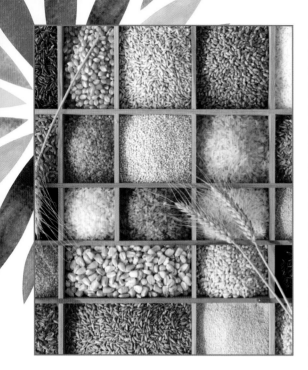

oats, corn (that means popcorn!), rice, and rye. The easiest way to tell whether a product is whole grain is to check the label and simply make sure the first word you see on it is "whole." Ingredients are listed on food products in order of weight, so if the first ingredient listed is a whole grain, then you're all set. Beware of products labeled as 100 percent Wheat, Multigrain, All-Natural, or Stone Ground. These may sound good, but they can be deceptive. Just because a product is 100 percent wheat doesn't mean the flour is whole wheat. Multigrain simply means there are two or more types of grain included, but it also doesn't say anything about whether they are whole. All-natural is practically meaningless, and shouldn't be confused with organic or whole grain. Stone ground flour is coarsely ground on a stone mill, but it also is not necessarily whole grain unless it's labeled as such.

day have been shown to have lower levels of risk factors for stroke, heart disease, diabetes, and cancers of the digestive system. Whole grains provide important nutrients, a rich supply of disease-fighting antioxidants, and plenty of fiber.

But that's not all. Whole grains are digested far more slowly than refined grains. This helps prevent insulin spikes as well as the crashes that lead to food cravings, drowsiness, and mood swings. By switching over to whole grains from refined grains, you're protecting your long-term health as well. Eating whole grains daily can help prevent diabetes and metabolic syndrome.

Whole grains include wheat, barley,

Whole grains can be part of your breakfast in the form of oatmeal, granola, or a muffin. They can be incorporated into your lunch and snacks in a variety of ways. And you can serve whole grains as a side dish with dinners, too.

**Milk and dairy products** play an important role in a healthy lifestyle. Dairy products are an excellent source of calcium, a mineral that is vital to your body's ability to build healthy bones and teeth as well as maintain many of its basic functions. Much of the milk available in North American grocery stores is also fortified with vitamin D. Making low-fat dairy products part of your daily diet may help prevent the development of insulin resistance and reduce the risk of developing type 2 diabetes.

Because whole milk is high in saturated fats, we recommend avoiding it in favor of skim milk, or else only consuming it in moderation. One cup of whole milk contains five grams of saturated fat; drinking whole milk on a regular basis can lead to higher levels of LDL cholesterol. The lactose contained in cheese and yogurt is also more easily digested than in milk, so

you may prefer these foods as the source of your dairy consumption.

**Seafood** is a staple of Mediterranean diets, for good reason. Seafood is a veritable gold mine of concentrated nutrients and minerals. Fish has very little saturated fat, and instead is rich in exactly the kind of monounsaturated fats and oils that have been shown to be so important to shedding belly fat, improving long-term cardiovascular health, and preventing diabetes. Fish is also rich in polyunsaturated fats, which remain liquid even when refrigerated. And while some kinds of shellfish do contain cholesterol, they're so low in saturated fats that they are unlikely to increase levels of cholesterol in the bloodstream. Fish and shellfish are also loaded with

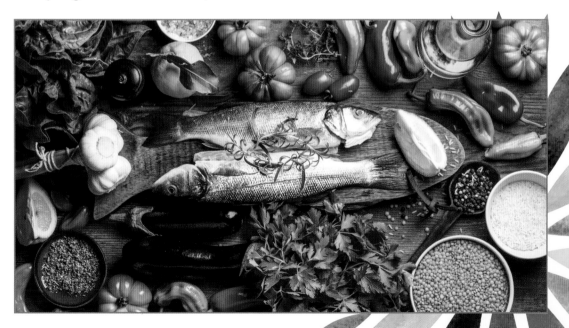

protein, but contain fewer calories per serving than red meat.

Eating fish three times a week or more can help to significantly reduce your risk of heart disease. The omega-3 fatty acids with which seafood is loaded help make blood platelets less likely to clot, lower inflammation in the arterial walls, and reduce levels of triglycerides in the bloodstream, all of which are risk factors for cardiovascular disease.

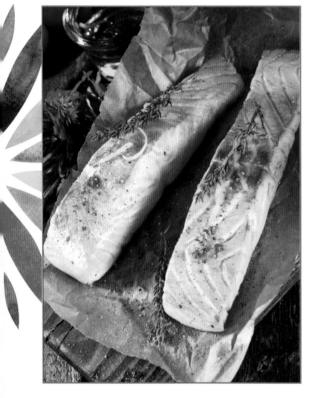

Eating more seafood also reduces the risk of stroke considerably, in particular ischemic stroke, which is brought on by blood clots. Regularly eating seafood rich in omega-3 fatty acids may also help to protect against age-related memory loss.

Certain types of fish are more susceptible to carrying pollutants, and should be avoided if you cannot find organically farm-raised varieties. These include tuna, shark, mackerel, and swordfish, all of which can accumulate dangerous levels of mercury in their tissues. Freshwater fish is typically not as susceptible to these kinds of pollutants, but you should make sure you know where your fish is coming from, and buy locally whenever possible.

Buy from a busy fish counter—the high turnover is an excellent way to ensure that the fish you are getting is fresh. When buying whole fish, avoid any fish with cloudy eyes or graying gills, and make sure the skin is bright with tight scales. When buying filets, avoid any that are discolored or that have gaps in the skin. Avoid filets that have a strong fishy odor, and buy those that smell briny and fresh.

**Red meat** is an excellent source of protein, which is vital to your body's proper functioning for a number of reasons. Protein is the basic unit of life, and without it your body couldn't build new cells or maintain existing ones. The proteins in red meat also function as a building

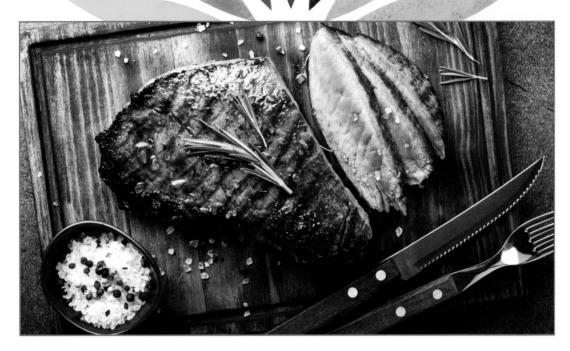

block for bones, muscles, cartilage, skin, and blood cells. They're also integral to your body's ability to produce enzymes, hormones, and vitamins. Proteins are essential to repairing tissues and cell walls, and some kinds of protein even help ward off infections and strengthen the immune system. Red meat contains selenium, a trace mineral that is critical to maintaining a healthy immune system.

The proteins found in red meat are also one of the things that help you feel full after you've eaten a meal. Your body takes longer to digest proteins than certain kinds of carbohydrates, so you won't get food cravings an hour after you've eaten. If you control your portions of fats and carbs by making one-

quarter of your meal lean protein, you'll be less likely to overindulge on less filling foods. Eating foods rich in proteins can also help you burn calories faster. That's because it takes more energy to break down and metabolize protein, which allows your body to burn more calories than when it is digesting fats and carbohydrates.

Red meat also helps protect you from losing muscle mass. Losing muscle mass will cause your metabolism to slow down, which can make it much harder to continue to lose weight. While strength training and an active lifestyle are very important to building muscle mass, what you consume will also affect your ability to maintain it as well.

## FOODS TO AVOID OR EAT IN SMALL PORTIONS

Now that we've covered all of the delicious things you can eat, let's look at which foods you will need to avoid or else eat in small portions only. These are foods that are rich in the bad kinds of fat—saturated and trans fats. Eating too much of either will increase the levels of LDL cholesterol and total cholesterol in your bloodstream.

**Saturated fats** do not necessarily have to be completely avoided, but for the most part you are better off finding alternatives to them or else only eating them in small portions. Saturated fat is higher in processed foods than in fresh foods. In general, it's better to avoid processed meats such as bologna and salami or only eat them occasionally and in small portions. Choose artisanal cheeses over processed cheese, and avoid American cheese slices altogether. Even then, try to eat only small amounts of cheese. Dairy-based desserts, like ice cream or mascarpone, contain saturated fats,

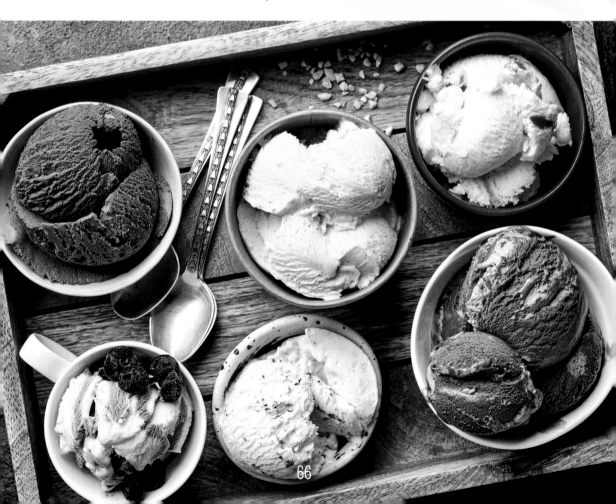

but not so much that you have to swear off dessert forever. But when you do eat dairy-based desserts, practice portion control and try not to eat them more than once a week at the most. Butter is far better than margarine, but it still contains a high amount of saturated fats. It's generally better to substitute olive oil for butter, but it's all right to treat yourself to a slice of buttered toast every now and then.

The good news about foods rich in saturated fat is that you don't have to cut them out of your diet entirely. That means that if any of the foods mentioned are among your favorites, they can be a great incentive to look forward to after you've met certain goals.

**Trans fats** and the foods that contain them are the ones that you should be steering clear of completely. This is not easy at first, because the versatility of trans fats has made them extremely popular with food manufacturers. Trans fats, or partially hydrogenated fats and oils, are in the vast majority of processed foods, fried and battered foods, and many frozen foods. But hydrogenated fats are terrible for your long-term cardiovascular health. They increase the levels of LDL and total cholesterol in the bloodstream while lowering the

levels of HDL cholesterol. Trans fats are incredibly destructive when you are trying to lose belly fat.

Remember to check the labels on the food products you're buying. Stay away from any that contain trans fats, hydrogenated fats, and partially hydrogenated fats. While you may not be able to completely cut trans fats out of your diet, you should be able to limit your daily intake of them to fewer than two grams per day. The following foods contain very high levels of trans fats and should be avoided:

**Margarine** was long believed to be the "healthy" alternative to natural butter, until we discovered that it's absolutely loaded with trans fats. Nowadays we know that it's better to avoid margarine altogether.

**Fried foods** are typically prepared in partially hydrogenated vegetable oil, which loads them up with trans fats. Sautee or pan-fry dishes in olive oil, and avoid fried foods when eating out. Eschew doughnuts altogether, since they're full of empty calories and almost always fried.

**Shortening** contains hydrogenated or partially hydrogenated fats, and it's used by a lot of fast food restaurants to prepare fried foods.

It also shows up regularly in baked goods such as pies, doughnuts, and cakes. Avoid shortening.

**Cake mixes** and store-bought frosting are convenient when you're planning a birthday party, but they are high in trans fats and empty calories. The best alternative is to bake a cake from scratch—you'll find that it's not difficult and can be a lot of fun!

**Refrigerated cookie dough** is also a convenient alternative to baking cookies from scratch, but like store-bought cake mixes and frosting, it's often loaded with trans fats. Fortunately, cookies are even easier to make from scratch than cake, and you can make sure you're using whole grain flour and organic

ingredients, too!

**Pie crusts** are made with shortening (see above) and butter. One slice of pie usually contains enough saturated and trans fats for nearly a week's worth of your recommended intake! You can make alternative pie crusts from scratch with whole grain flour and natural vegetable oil that taste just as good.

**Frozen dinners** aren't always bad, but you'll have to carefully read the nutrition information label before you buy them. Many frozen dinners, especially those that are breaded, have plenty of trans fats. Choose frozen dinners with minimally processed foods, or opt for frozen vegetables that you season at home.

**Non-dairy creamer** may appear to be an innocuous way to quickly add flavor to your morning coffee, but it's full of trans fats. Try 1 percent milk or evaporated skim milk instead.

**Microwave popcorn** is usually loaded with salt and artificial "butter flavor" that is full of trans fats. Fortunately, making popcorn the old-fashioned way is a fun and easy alternative, and it's good for you!

Beyond avoiding trans fats and reducing your intake of saturated fats, there are a few more general

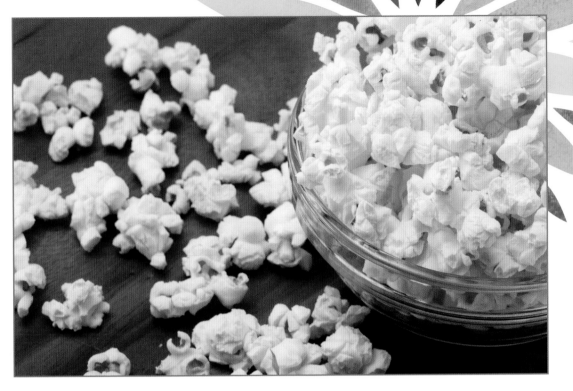

guidelines to eating healthy. First, it's better to avoid processed foods in favor of those that are as close to their natural state as possible. If you must purchase a processed food product, carefully read the label to make sure it is low in sodium and saturated fats and does not contain trans fats. Soft drinks and flavored drinks should be avoided as much as possible. Most soft drinks are full of high fructose corn syrup, which is not good for your long-term health. Instead, make iced tea, or slice a cucumber into a pitcher of water for a refreshing, delicious drink.

## ADDING IN OILS

We talked a little bit about the importance of oils earlier. Here's some more specific information as you choose oils that you can use to cook and add flavor to your foods.

As discussed earlier, olive oil was central to the discovery that the Mediterranean diet has beneficial effects on long-term health. Olive oil reduces inflammation throughout the entire body, reduces rates of heart disease, and helps decrease your total cholesterol and LDL cholesterol levels in the bloodstream.

Canola oil is high in polyunsaturated

fats, which are not quite as good as MUFAs for your heart health and cholesterol levels, but still far better than saturated fats. Canola oil has less saturated fat than any other oil commonly used in North America. It has been linked to lower blood pressure, cholesterol, and arterial inflammation. Canola oil is also high in alpha-linoleic acid, one of the omega-3 fatty acids that your body can't produce on its own.

Flaxseed oil has been a staple of the Mediterranean diet for centuries and is becoming increasingly popular in North America because of its health benefits. Flaxseed oil also contains alpha-linoleic acid, and there is solid evidence that making it part of your daily diet can help lower LDL and total cholesterol levels in the bloodstream. Flaxseed oil also has a moderate effect on triglyceride levels, and it may improve kidney function and relieve symptoms related to menopause.

Peanut oil is full of monounsaturated fats and polyunsaturated fats,

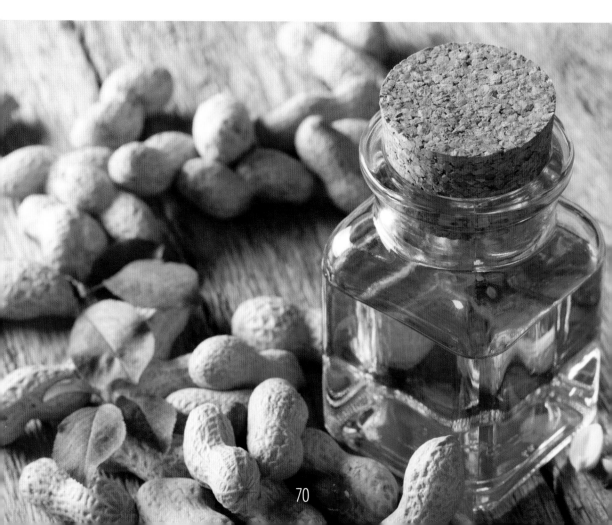

so it's highly recommended that you incorporate it into your diet. Peanut oil has the added benefit of being absolutely loaded with antioxidants, particularly vitamin E, which helps protect your cellular health by neutralizing free radicals. This can help lower your risk of certain cancers and heart disease, which are thought to be linked to an excess of free radicals in the system. Peanut oil is calorie-rich, so try to consume it in moderation.

Safflower oil is another rich source of MUFAs. It provides a quarter of your daily recommended intake of vitamin E, and it has been linked to regulating blood glucose levels and reducing inflammation in diabetic patients. Safflower oil is also amazingly versatile in the kitchen. It has a high smoke point, so you can use it to sauté and fry many different dishes, and it has a mild flavor, which makes it great for salad dressing and marinades.

Sesame oil is bursting with antioxidants, making it a favorite health food. It's great for your skin and hair, and it has antibacterial and anti-inflammatory properties as well. Studies have shown that consuming it on a regular basis can help lower blood pressure as well as glucose and sodium levels in the bloodstream. The best part? Sesame oil is simply delicious! It has a rich, almost nutty flavor, and a little bit goes a long way.

Soybean oil is great to use— in moderation. While it is full of omega-3 fatty acids and polyunsaturated fats, it has more total fat per serving than any of the other oils mentioned here. That means that it is an excellent source of cholesterol-lowering unsaturated fats and a great substitute for unhealthy saturated fat, but you should avoid consuming too much of it.

Sunflower oil is another great source of linoleic acid, vitamin E, and polyunsaturated fats. It's also cholesterol- and sodium-free, and particularly low in saturated fats. Refined sunflower oil has a high smoke point, which makes it excellent for sautéing, and a mild flavor, which makes it great as a salad dressing or marinade.

By trying these different oils, you'll soon find which ones you prefer to use in the kitchen. Some are more versatile than others; some have richer flavors that you may prefer to more mild oils. No matter which of these oils you decide to add to your diet, you can enjoy knowing that they're not just delicious and adaptable to lots of different recipes —they're great for your long-term health!

**Butter**, unlike liquid oils, has a lot of saturated fat, as much as 58 grams per stick. It also contains monounsaturated fat, about 24 grams per stick, and around 800 calories. So while it isn't nearly as bad as margarine, which is loaded with trans fats and saturated fat, it's not nearly as good as any of the oils recommended above, either. You can treat yourself to moderate amounts of butter every once in a while. Make sure you are choosing unsalted butter, and if you can, opt for "grass-fed" butter. Butter from grass-fed cows is much richer and more flavorful, and it's likely sourced from smaller farms, which means it will be of better quality.

## THE ROLE OF SALT

"Salt" and "sodium" are words that are often used interchangeably when discussing diet, but they are not the same. Sodium is an element that is a component of table salt; the other component is chlorine. Sodium is found naturally in the majority of foods, and salt is the source of most of the sodium in our diet. Sodium is an important part of our diet. It promotes healthy nerve function; without sodium, our nerves would not be able to transmit signals to one another. We wouldn't be able to contract our muscles or maintain our heartbeat. Sodium is also crucial to our body's ability to maintain its internal pH.

But salt also plays another important role: It helps to maintain our body's fluid balance. *Osmolarity* is the scientific word that describes the ratio of body fluids to solutes, the substances dissolved in those body fluids. If there is a lot of variation in the body's osmolarity, it can cause cells to swell up or shrivel, and in the process damage or even destroy cellular structure and disrupt normal cellular function. For example, if you become dehydrated, you lose a lot of water, but retain solute (as sodium), and the osmolarity of your bodily fluids goes up. Your kidneys play a major role in balancing the absorption and excretion of water and sodium into your bloodstream. This is the main way your body is able to regulate its osmolarity.

In the majority of bodily fluids, sodium is the main solute, so it is the substance that determines the osmolarity of the body. When we eat a lot of salty foods, our kidneys notice the change in osmolarity and signal the body to retain water in order to maintain a balanced osmolarity. This temporary conservation of fluids causes us to hold on to excess water weight, look bloated and puffy, and feel tired.

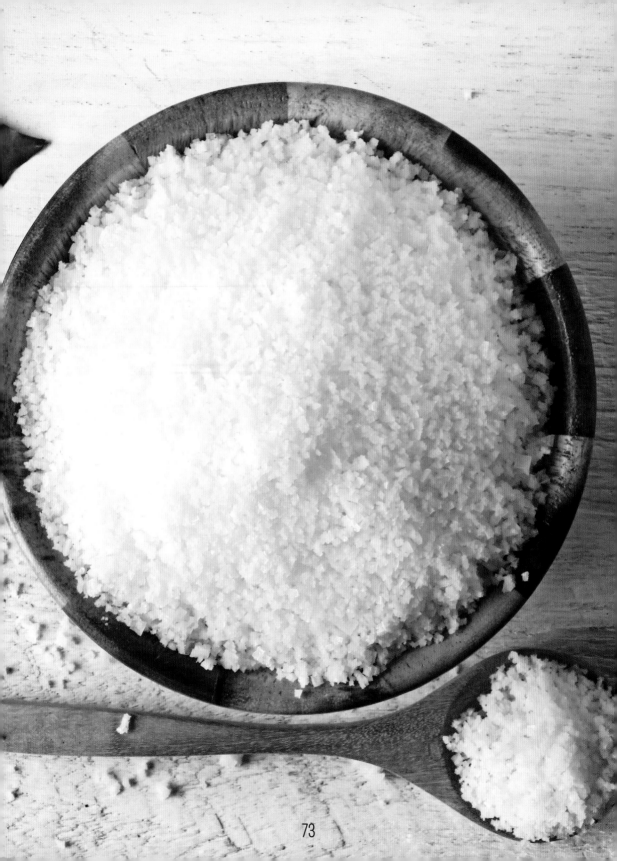

Does this mean you should cut salt out of your diet entirely? Not at all. Cutting back on salt and increasing the amount of water you drink on a daily basis will go a long way to bringing your body back to a balanced osmolarity. You'll also find that after only a short amount of time using less salt, your palate will adjust accordingly, and you will soon be able to notice smaller amounts of salt in your meals.

This will actually allow you to enjoy meals more. When your dishes aren't overwhelmed by saltiness, the complexity of the other flavor profiles in them will be allowed to flourish. That is the culinary purpose of salt: It's meant to bring out the flavors in the dish, rather than overpower them. If you tend to impulsively reach for the salt shaker, try tasting your dishes before you salt them. You'll probably find that most of them need very little salt, if any. And try switching to kosher salt. It has larger grains than other kinds of table salt, so it tastes saltier and you can use less of it to get the same flavor.

You can also cut down on the amount of sodium in your diet by eating more fresh fruits and vegetables rather than buying canned. If you do use canned vegetables, look for "Low Sodium" or

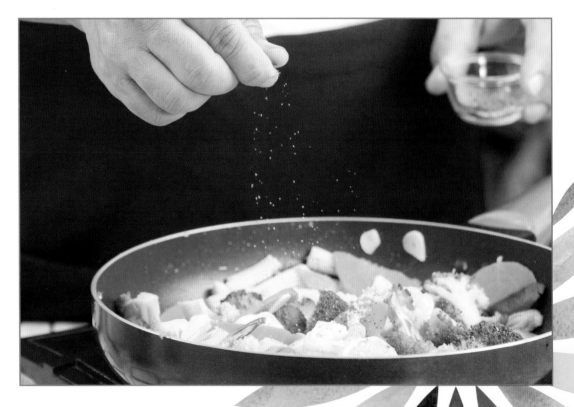

"No Salt Added" on the label.

Instead of buying instant potatoes, use fresh ones. Buy fresh or frozen fish instead of canned or dried, and avoid processed meats like bologna or salami in favor of deli sliced meat. Some of the best tools that can help to make it easier to reduce your sodium intake are on your spice rack. Many of the most common spices and seasonings we use on a regular basis are loaded with compounds that can help regulate your blood sugar or boost your metabolism. Seasonings and spices also have very few calories, so you can add them to your heart's desire to add variety and flavor to your meals. The most ordinary dish can suddenly become haute cuisine with the right combination of spices, so you'll never endure a dull minute in the kitchen again.

The following spices are particularly useful for boosting your metabolism, and decreasing chronic inflammation:

**Black pepper** is one of the most common spices; it's usually right next to your salt shaker. But what you might not know about it is that its flavor comes from a compound called *piperine*, which has been shown to actually inhibit the production of new fat cells. That means that incorporating more black pepper into your diet can help you lose more belly fat faster. Pepper is also rich in antioxidants and is an excellent digestive aid. To get the most out of your black pepper, purchase a pepper mill and buy whole black peppercorns. Grinding fresh pepper onto your dishes will enhance their flavors and may eventually have you foregoing the salt shaker altogether!

**Cinnamon** is a delicious, savory-sweet spice that can be added to desserts as well as main dishes such as curry or dry rubs. A little bit of cinnamon goes a long way, not only in terms of flavor but also in the health benefits it provides. Cinnamon has a complex molecule called methyl hydroxychalcone polymer, and studies have shown

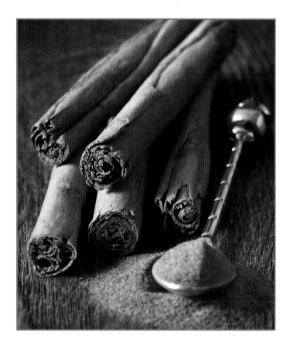

that this compound can improve your fat cells' insulin receptiveness. That means that consuming cinnamon will help prevent the

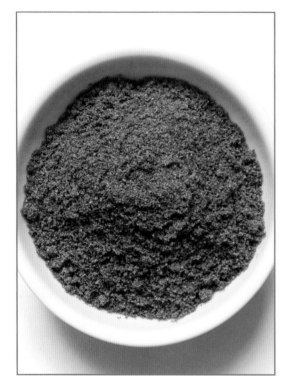

insulin crashes that lead to mood swings, irritability, and cravings.

**Cumin** has an almost nutty flavor to it, but it's best when it's paired with other spices, such as curry powder, cayenne, or garam masala. Cumin is perfect for tying the various spices in a dish together into a delicious, uniform combination of flavor. It's loaded with health benefits, too. It can help regulate blood sugar levels and alleviate stress by reducing the circulation of stress hormones like cortisol in the bloodstream. And cumin has very high concentrations of antioxidants that fight free radicals and help maintain long-term health. You can either buy whole cumin seeds or powdered cumin. Powdered cumin should be added to spice mixes, while cumin seeds can be lightly toasted and added to many different savory dishes.

**Garlic** isn't just one of the most pungent and delicious flavors to add to any dish, it's also one of the healthiest things you can incorporate into your diet. Garlic has been shown to lower total cholesterol and LDL cholesterol levels in the bloodstream, lower blood pressure, and decrease risk factors for heart disease and certain types of cancer. It also helps to maintain insulin levels in the bloodstream, which is critical to preventing the kinds of spikes or crashes that lead to mood swings, tiredness, and—you guessed it—food cravings. Garlic also has thermogenic properties, which means it takes more energy to digest it, helping you burn more calories and boost your metabolism when you incorporate it into your diet. You can buy garlic in many different forms, either as fresh bulbs, or peeled and minced in jars, or powdered and dried. The best health benefits (and the most flavor)

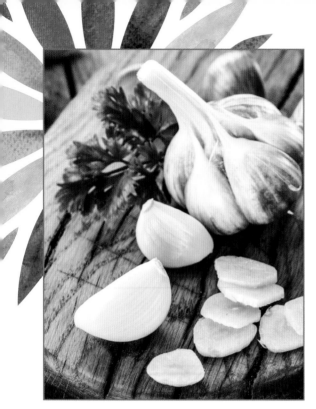

prevent certain types of cancer. Turmeric also helps to reduce blood sugar, and it protects against insulin resistance. By incorporating turmeric into your diet, you can reduce the levels of insulin, stress hormones like cortisol, and inflammation markers in the bloodstream.

Cooking with spices takes some trial and error to get it right, so don't be discouraged if you aren't successful right away. Try adding small amounts of these spices to your dishes at first, and as you grow more confident, you'll want to experiment by combining them to produce new flavor profiles. Once you're comfortable cooking with these five basic spices, you can start to explore others, such as ginger, garam masala, fennel, cloves, and coriander, all of which are also delicious and great for you.

## THE ROLE OF SUGAR

Many diets rule out sugar altogether, and often for good reason. But the fact is that there are different kinds of sugar, and they have different effects on your ability to lose belly fat and keep it off. Sugar is an important part of our diet—it provides energy that we need to get through the day, and the brain gets most of its functional energy by metabolizing glucose. Our ancestors

are in fresh garlic. You can add garlic to sautéed vegetables, soups, salad dressings, curries, marinades, and sauces, and add it to fish, poultry, and red meat to enhance natural flavors and create delicious meals.

**Turmeric** is a South Asian spice that has been used for centuries in Indian cuisine as a flavoring and coloring agent. Turmeric is related to ginger, and it has a bright yellow color. It's slightly bitter by itself, but when incorporated into a spice mix with cumin and garam masala, it adds an almost buttery mustard quality that is as unique as it is delicious. Turmeric has antioxidant and anti-inflammatory properties, and a diet rich in turmeric may even needed sugar to survive, and it could be difficult to come by when we were hunter-gatherers, which is one of the reasons we've developed such a love of sweet foods. But refined sugar, which is a relatively new development in our diets, is not only much purer than the sugars found in natural sources like fruits and vegetables, but it's much more common as well.

Because of sugar's purity and availability, it's easy to consume far too much sugar today. This can wreak havoc on our health in many ways. It can cause cavities. It can lead to insulin resistance, metabolic syndrome, and type 2 diabetes. Too much sugar can interfere with brain function, cause mood swings and irritability, and lead to poor decision-making. Be careful to watch your intake of two kinds of sugars: simple sugars and refined carbohydrates.

**Simple sugar** is what's in your sugar bowl. Simple sugars include basic white sugar, powdered (or confectioner's) sugar, sugar cubes, and brown sugar, which is basic white sugar with molasses added to it. Whenever you add simple

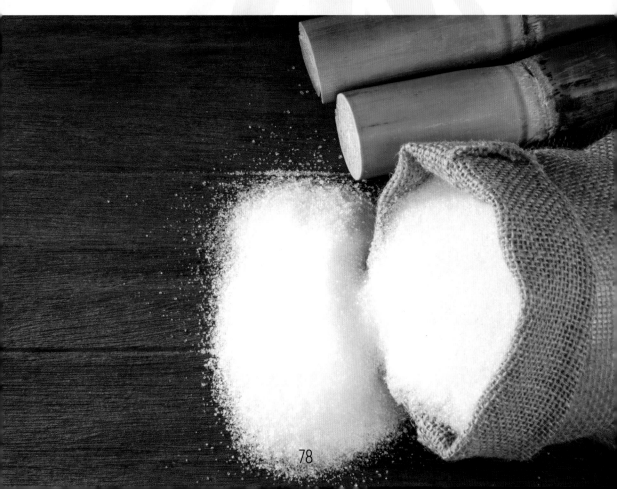

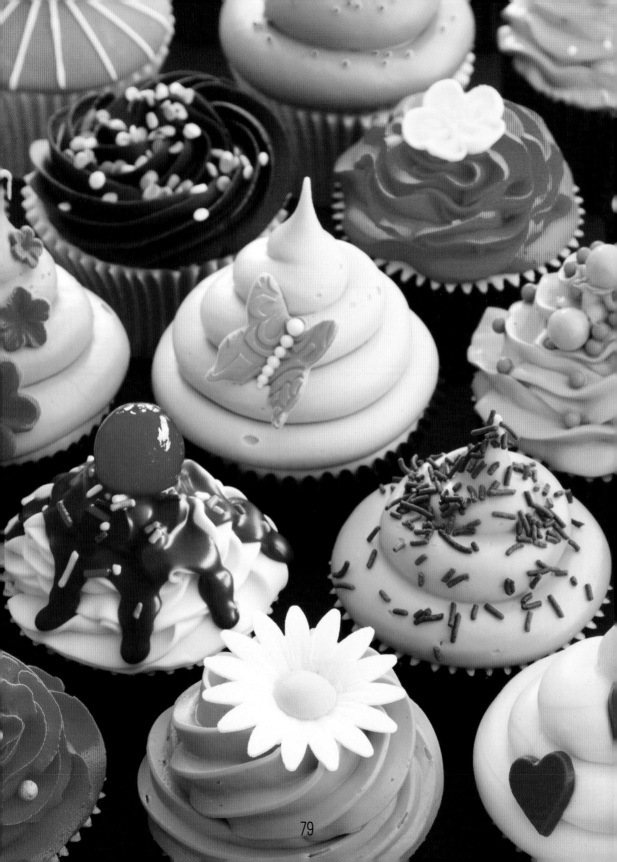

sugars to your tea or coffee, sprinkle sugar on your cereal or eat sugary desserts or sweets, you're giving your body a huge influx of simple sugars. This is what can cause spikes and crashes in blood sugar levels, leading to massive fluctuation of insulin levels. Avoid simple sugars as much as possible. Steer clear of sweetened beverages, opting for water, unsweetened iced teas, or seltzer water instead.

**Refined carbohydrates** are a kind of sugar that is found in foods made with enriched and white flour. Unlike whole grain flours, the carbohydrates in these flours are digested very rapidly, which again leads to spikes in blood sugar and insulin levels. Avoid refined carbohydrates in favor of whole grains, which take longer to metabolize, helping you avoid sugar spikes, crashes, and cravings.

Fruits are an excellent source of the sugars your body needs to function, but they come in natural, unprocessed packages that don't cause the kind of blood sugar spikes that cause you to retain belly fat. Fruits are also loaded with antioxidants, fiber, and nutrients that help you maintain your long-term health. Many fruits help fight insulin resistance, reduce chronic inflammation, and lower stress hormone levels in the bloodstream.

Of course, that doesn't mean you should immediately start eating as much fruit as possible. While fruit is good for you and can help you fight belly fat, the fact that it contains natural sugars means that if you eat too much of it, you may wind up actually promoting weight gain. Remember to keep your portions moderate and include it as part of a balanced diet.

Are you ready to put your new food knowledge to use?

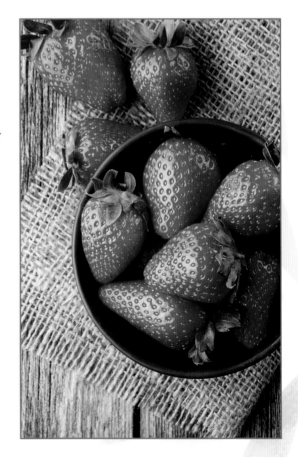

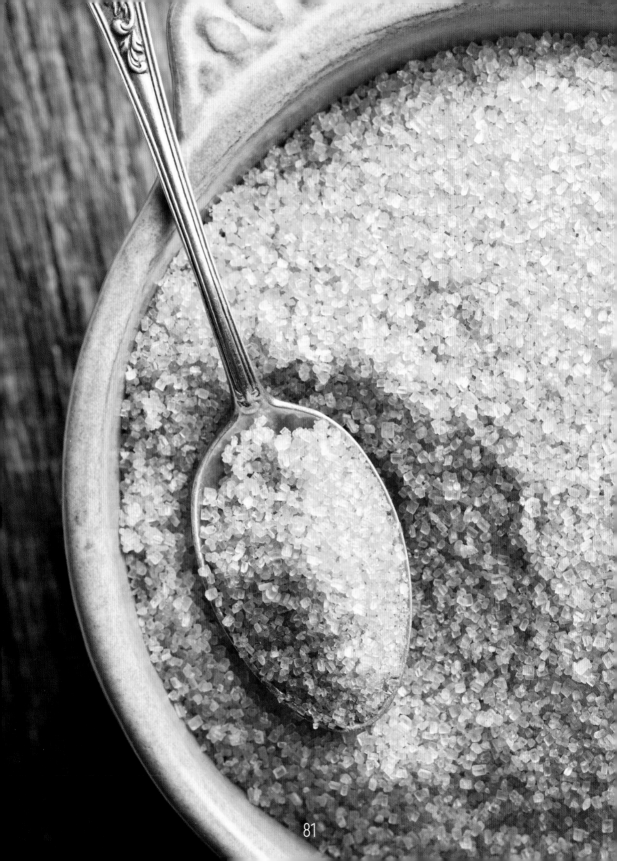

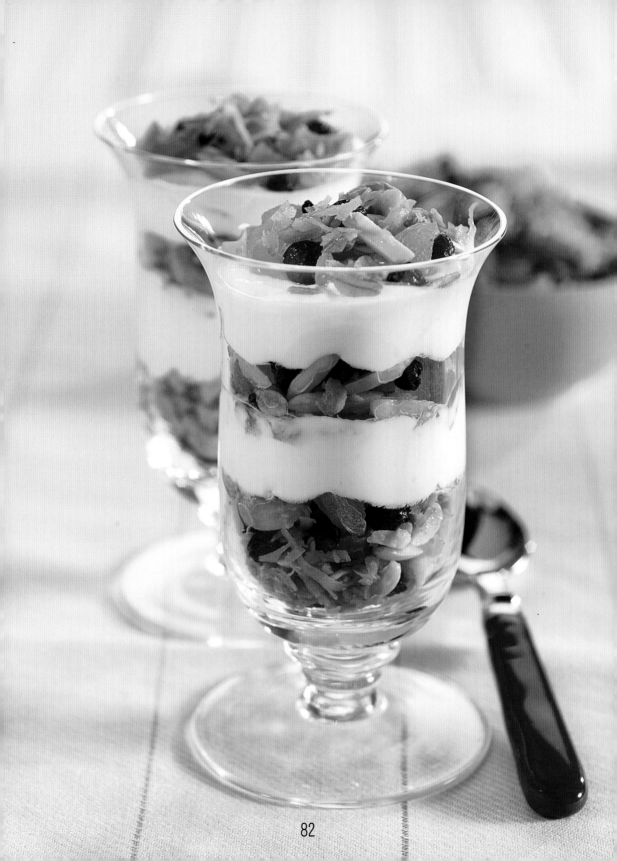

# CHUNKY FRUITY
# HOMEMADE GRANOLA

2 cups old-fashioned oats

1⅓ cups raw slivered almonds

1 cup shredded coconut

3 tablespoons butter

¼ cup honey

1 cup dried apricots, chopped

¾ cup dried cranberries

¾ cup dried tart cherries

½ cup dried blueberries

½ cup roasted unsalted cashew pieces

1. Preheat oven to 300°F. Line baking sheet with foil or parchment paper.

2. Combine oats, almonds, and coconut in large bowl. Place butter in small microwavable bowl; microwave on HIGH for 30 to 45 seconds or until melted. Whisk in honey until blended. Pour butter mixture over oat mixture; toss to coat. Spread on prepared baking sheet.

3. Bake 20 to 25 minutes or until golden, stirring once or twice during baking. Cool mixture on baking sheet on wire rack.

4. Combine apricots, cranberries, cherries, blueberries and cashews in large bowl. Crumble cooled oat mixture into fruit mixture; stir until blended.

**MAKES ABOUT 8 CUPS**

Serving Suggestions: Layer the granola with a cup of yogurt for a quick breakfast parfait. It can be served as a snack on its own, or as part of a dessert sprinkled over ice cream or frozen yogurt. Keep it stored in an airtight container to maintain its crispiness.

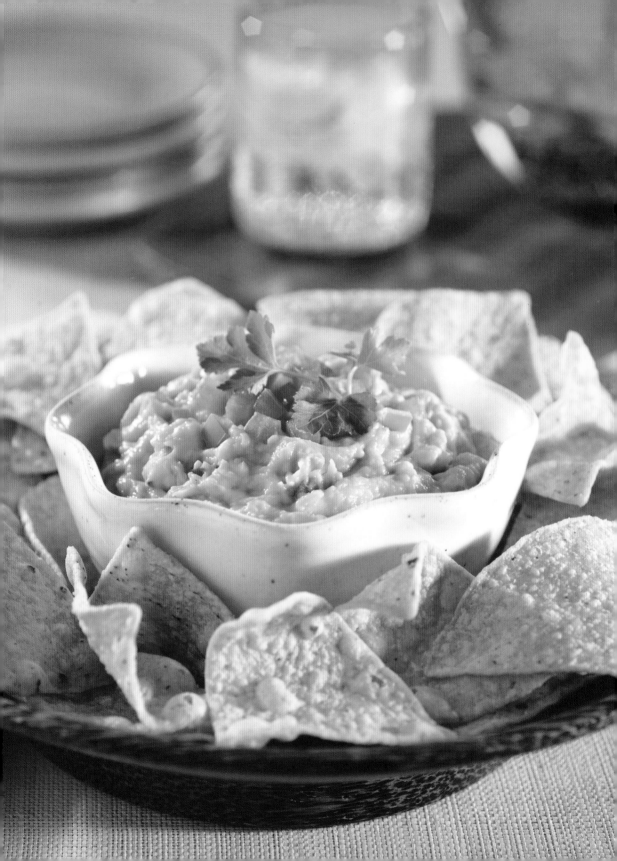

# GUACAMOLE

2 large avocados

¼ cup finely chopped tomato, plus additional for garnish

2 tablespoons fresh lime juice or lemon juice

2 tablespoons grated onion with juice

½ teaspoon salt

¼ teaspoon hot pepper sauce

Black pepper

**1.** Place avocados in medium bowl; mash coarsely with fork. Stir in ¼ cup tomato, lime juice, onion with juice, salt, hot pepper sauce and black pepper; mix well.

**2.** Serve immediately or cover and refrigerate up to 2 hours. Garnish with additional tomato.

**MAKES 2 CUPS**

Tip: To ripen firm avocados, store them in a loosely closed paper bag at room temperature for a few days.

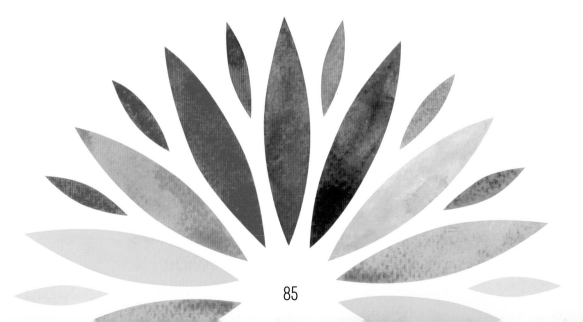

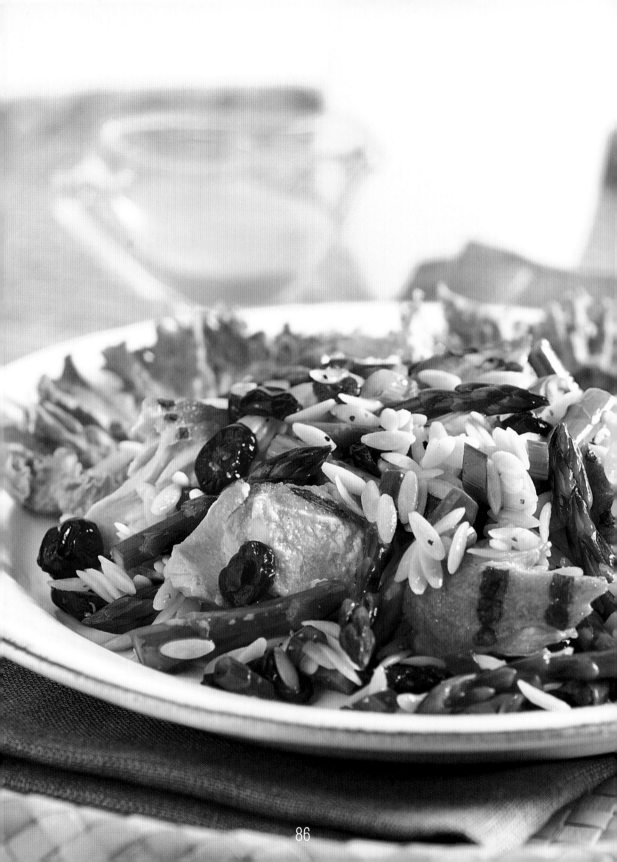

# SALMON, ASPARAGUS AND ORZO SALAD

1 (8-ounce) salmon fillet

1 cup uncooked orzo pasta

8 ounces asparagus, cooked and cut into 2-inch pieces (about 1½ cups)

½ cup dried cranberries

¼ cup sliced green onions

3 tablespoons extra virgin olive oil

1 tablespoon white wine vinegar

1½ teaspoons Dijon mustard

½ teaspoon salt

⅛ teaspoon black pepper

1. Prepare grill for direct cooking. Oil grid.

2. Grill salmon over medium heat about 10 minutes per inch of thickness or until opaque in center. Remove to plate; cool 10 minutes. Flake salmon into bite-size pieces.

3. Meanwhile, cook orzo according to package directions; drain and cool.

4. Combine salmon, orzo, asparagus, cranberries and green onions in large bowl. Whisk oil, vinegar, mustard, salt and pepper in small bowl until well blended. Pour over salmon mixture; toss gently to coat. Refrigerate 30 minutes to 1 hour.

**MAKES 4 TO 6 SERVINGS**

# HOT AND SOUR SOUP
# WITH BOK CHOY AND TOFU

1 tablespoon dark sesame oil

4 ounces fresh shiitake mushrooms, stems finely chopped, caps thinly sliced

2 cloves garlic, minced

2 cups mushroom broth or vegetable broth

1 cup plus 2 tablespoons cold water, divided

2 tablespoons reduced-sodium soy sauce

1½ tablespoons rice vinegar or white wine vinegar

¼ teaspoon red pepper flakes

1½ tablespoons cornstarch

2 cups coarsely chopped bok choy leaves or napa cabbage

10 ounces silken extra firm tofu, well drained, cut into ½-inch cubes

1 green onion, thinly sliced

**1.** Heat oil in large saucepan over medium heat. Add mushrooms and garlic; cook and stir four minutes. Add broth, one cup water, soy sauce, vinegar and red pepper flakes; bring to a boil. Reduce heat to low; cook 5 minutes.

**2.** Whisk remaining 2 tablespoons water into cornstarch in small bowl until smooth. Stir into soup; cook 2 minutes or until thickened. Stir in bok choy; cook 2 to 3 minutes or until wilted. Stir in tofu; heat through. Sprinkle with green onion.

**MAKES 4 SERVINGS**

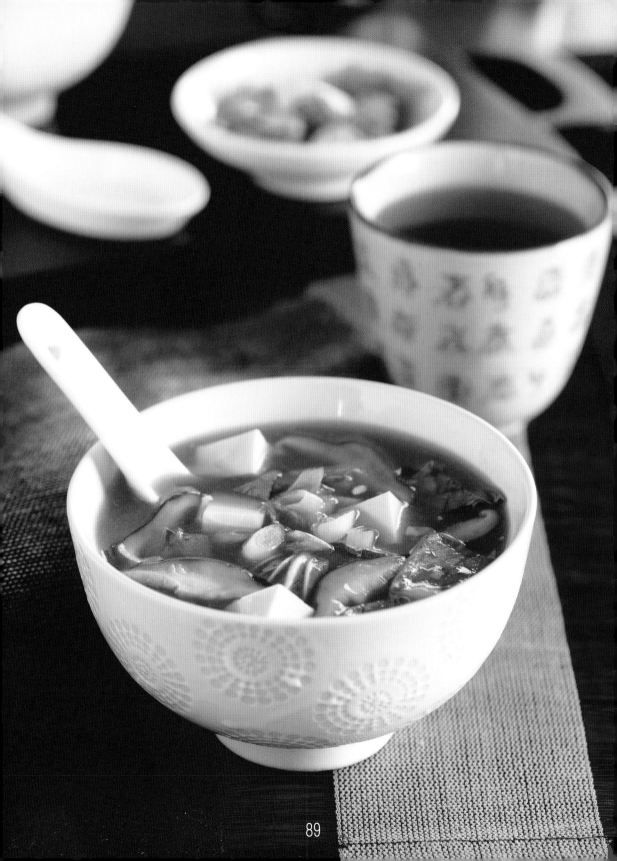

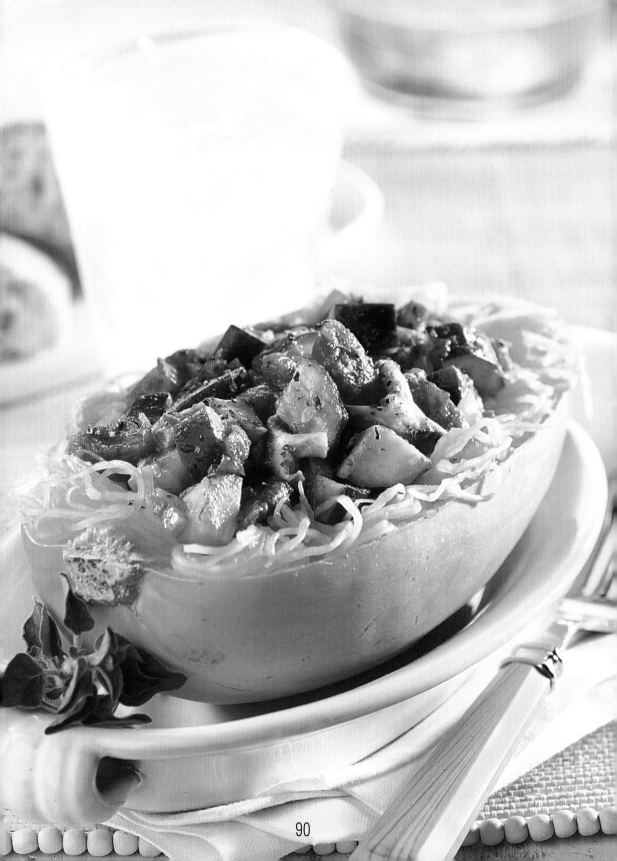

# SPICY RATATOUILLE
# WITH SPAGHETTI SQUASH

1 spaghetti squash (2 pounds)

2 tablespoons olive oil

1 small onion, finely chopped

1 clove garlic, minced

1 small eggplant, diced

1 small zucchini, diced

1 cup coarsely chopped mushrooms, preferably oyster or shiitake

1 can (about 14 ounces) diced tomatoes

1 tablespoon canned chipotle pepper in adobo sauce, minced

½ teaspoon dried oregano

½ teaspoon salt

¼ teaspoon black pepper

Grated Parmesan cheese (optional)

**1.** Pierce squash skin with fork or paring knife several times; place on microwavable plate. Cover loosely with plastic wrap; microwave on HIGH 12 to 13 minutes, turning after 6 minutes. (Squash is fully cooked when fork pierces skin and flesh easily.) Set aside to cool 5 minutes.

**2.** When squash is cool enough to handle, cut in half lengthwise. Scoop out and discard seeds. Separate squash into strands with fork. Measure 2 cups; cover and set aside. Save the empty squash shell halves, if desired.*

**3.** While squash cooks, heat oil in large skillet. Add onion and garlic; cook and stir over medium-high heat one minute. Add eggplant, zucchini and mushrooms; cook and stir heat 5 minutes or until vegetables are lightly browned. Stir in tomatoes, chipotle pepper, oregano, salt and pepper; cook over medium heat 3 to 5 minutes or until slightly thickened and heated through.

**4.** Spread squash on serving plate; top with ratatouille. Sprinkle with cheese, if desired. Serve immediately.

*For a unique presentation, serve the ratatouille in the empty squash shell halves.

**MAKES 4 SERVINGS**

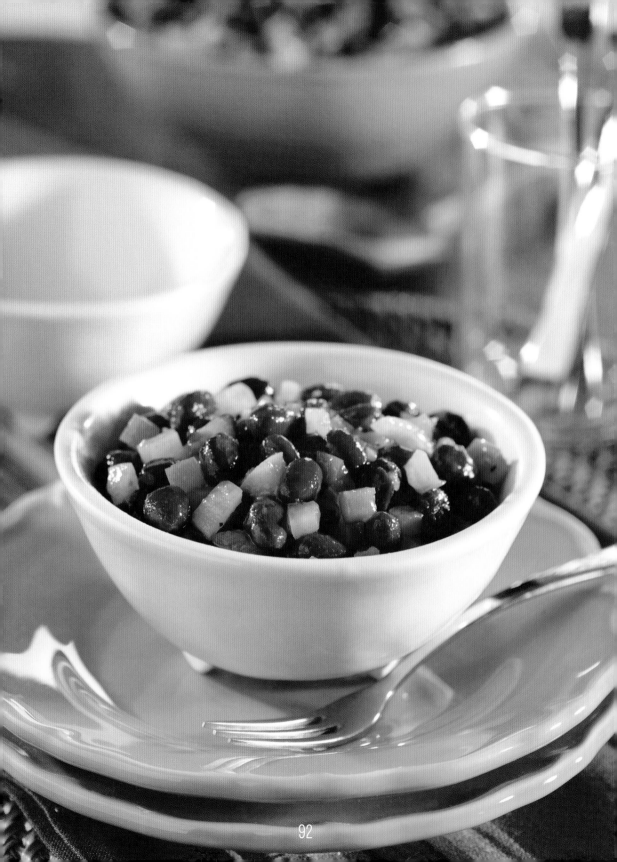

# CONFETTI BLACK BEANS

1 cup dried black beans, rinsed and sorted

3 cups water

1 can (about 14 ounces) reduced-sodium chicken broth

1 bay leaf

1 tablespoon olive oil

1 medium onion, chopped

¼ cup chopped red bell pepper

¼ cup chopped yellow bell pepper

2 cloves garlic, minced

1 jalapeño pepper,* finely chopped

1 large tomato, seeded and chopped

½ teaspoon salt

⅛ teaspoon black pepper

Hot pepper sauce (optional)

*Jalapeño peppers can sting and irritate the skin, so wear rubber gloves when handling peppers and do not touch your eyes.

1. Place beans in large bowl; add water. Soak the beans for 8 hours or overnight.

2. Drain beans. Combine beans and broth in large saucepan; bring to a boil over high heat. Add bay leaf. Reduce heat to low; cover and simmer 1½ hours or until beans are tender.

3. Heat oil in large nonstick skillet over medium heat. Add onion, bell peppers, garlic and jalapeño pepper; cook and stir 8 to 10 minutes or until onion is translucent. Add tomato, salt and black pepper; cook for 5 minutes.

4. Add onion mixture to beans; cook 15 to 20 minutes. Remove and discard bay leaf. Serve with hot pepper sauce, if desired.

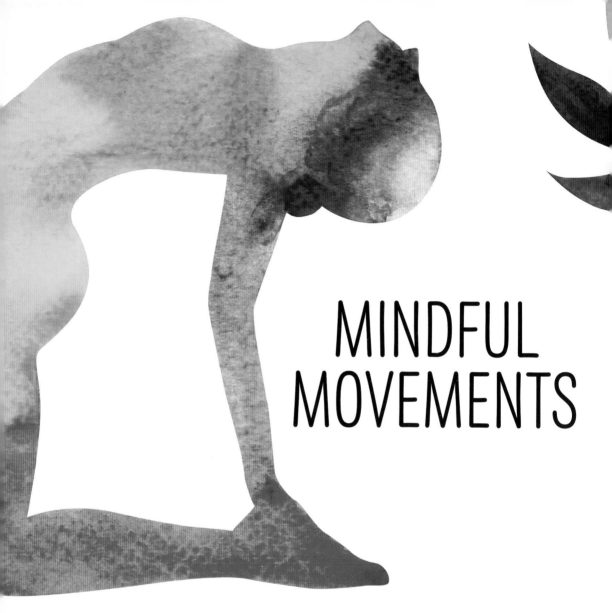

# MINDFUL MOVEMENTS

## FROM MIND TO BODY

Mindfulness can reduce stress, lift spirits, and improve general health. But when you incorporate mindfulness with exercise, the combination can do wonders for your wellbeing.

It can be hard to carve out time for exercise. When you spend eight hours a day (or more) at your workplace, an hour getting ready for work in the morning, and another two to three hours commuting to and from work, half of your day is literally gone by the time you get

94

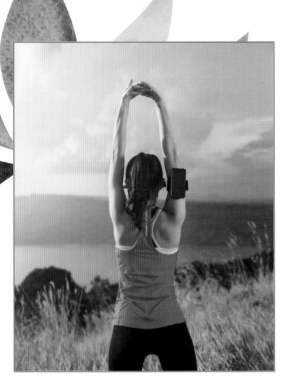

and risk factors for dozens of chronic diseases. Simply by increasing the amount of time you spend walking or standing as compared to how many hours a day you spend sitting has been shown to drastically reduce your chances of developing heart disease later in life. Increasing your daily activity can also improve memory and brain function and may help prevent neurological diseases like Alzheimer's.

Combining mindfulness with exercise can start with something as simple as walking meditation. Focus your attention on the movement of breath through the lungs, the action of the arms and legs as each step is taken, and the smells, sights, and sounds of the environment as you walk. Ultimately, such 'mindful movements' can encompass a variety of activities; the goal is to be aware of your body as you walk, run, cycle, lift, and stretch.

home. Then there's everything that needs to be done around the house, whether or not you have a family. Once you factor in everything you are obligated to take care of, there's precious little time for your own pursuits.

Yet daily activity has immediate and long-term effects. The immediate effects are pretty straightforward: You're burning calories, which means you're dropping pounds and getting fit. That's great all by itself.

But the long-term effects of daily activity are more profound. Just getting 10 or 20 minutes of cardio and weight training in each day can have incredible effects on your longevity, cardiovascular health,

In the rest of this chapter, you'll find step-by-step instructions and accompanying photographs for fitness ball exercises and yoga poses. These exercises and poses are not only accessible for most fitness levels, but they are also excellent opportunities to practice moving your body with mindful intention.

# BALL EXERCISES

Ball exercise routines are very low-impact and can be engaged in at whatever intensity level you are comfortable with. That means that you can scale up intensity at whatever pace works best for you. Fitness ball exercises can also be incorporated into your daily routine, especially if you spend a lot of time sitting. Just swap out your office chair for a large fitness ball, and you can do exercises while you work. Ball exercises are particularly great for building your core strength.

The basic ball workout is to simply sit on the ball with your shoulders back and your core engaged, and simply bounce! The key to this exercise is to bounce up rather than bounce down. Reach forward and back while you bounce, and vary bringing your arms in or out. Do this for about five minutes at a time over the course of the day. You'll be amazed by what a difference this simple routine will have!

For more involved ball exercises, you can try different positions and routines. You can walk your legs out until your shoulders rest on the ball and your knees are at a 90-degree angle. Extend your arms toward the ceiling, clasp your hands together, and engage your glutes. Walk your feet back as you move into a sitting position.

You can develop these exercises or make up your own that involve picking the ball up, bouncing on it in different ways, or using it as a support for other exercises. These exercises can also be made slightly more intensive by using three- or five-pound dumbbells to help tone your arm muscles while you engage your core. The most important thing is to pay attention to your breath as you complete each movement.

# PELVIC CIRCLES

This exercise is designed to enhance core strength and improve balance. Pelvic circles are low intensity and add no impact to the spine. This exercise is a challenge for those with balance issues, so use the ball with caution.

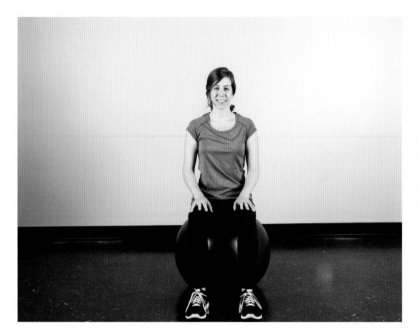

## STEP 1

Sit on a stability ball with feet flat on the floor, spine tall. Pull the abdominals in toward the spine.

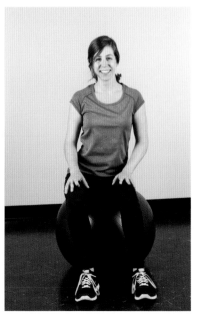
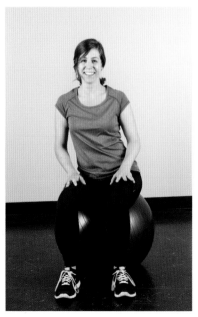

## STEP 2

Make a circular motion with the hips moving in a clockwise direction. Do 15 repetitions, then repeat going in the other direction.

# HIP EXTENSIONS

Hip extensions target the hips and legs, both important muscles for walking. Adding the stability ball engages the core muscles and adds a balance challenge to the exercise. This is a no-impact, moderate-intensity exercise.

## STEP 1

Lie flat on your back with ankles resting on a stability ball, legs straight.

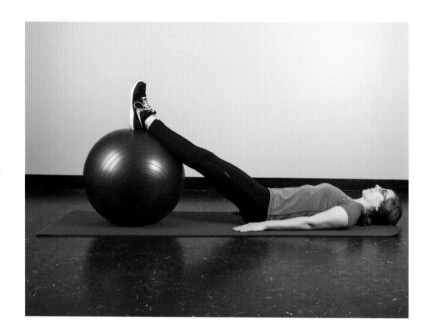

## STEP 2

Keeping legs straight and abdominals contracted, lift hips towards ceiling. Keep neck and shoulders relaxed.

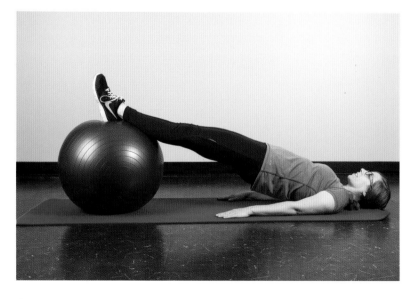

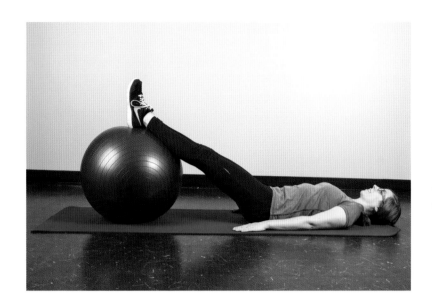

## STEP 3

Pause for one count at the top of the lift. With firm abdominals, lower the hips back to the floor. Do 10-15 repetitions.

# BACK EXTENSIONS

This exercise is a low-intensity back exercise that helps to improve posture and core strength. Back extensions are of moderate impact to the spine, so people with spinal stenosis should avoid this exercise.

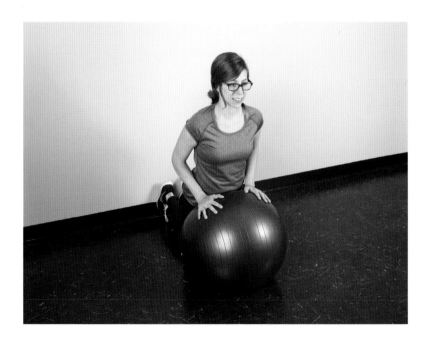

## STEP 1

Bring the ball to an area with a wall nearby. Kneel in front of the ball. Lean forward, placing abdominals on the ball.

## STEP 2

Straighten legs, securing feet against a wall.

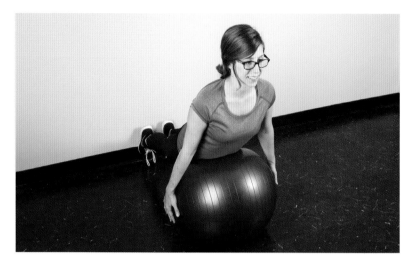

## STEP 3

Round the upper body forward so it is draped over the ball.

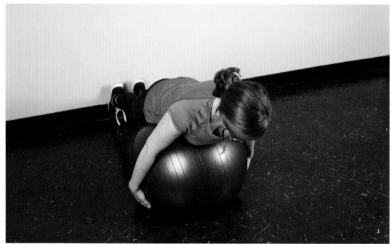

## STEP 4

Lift the head and shoulders up until upper body is in line with lower body. Do not extend beyond a straight spine. Do 10-15 repetitions.

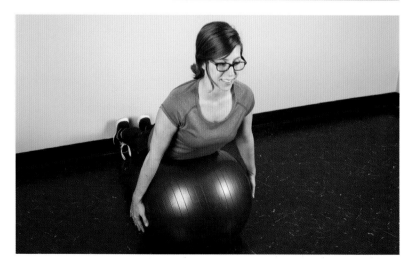

# WALL SQUAT

Wall squats are a moderate-intensity, moderate-impact exercise designed to strengthen the legs. This exercise also engages the core muscles. If knee pain is present, only squat halfway or to tolerance. Use caution if suffering from peripheral neuropathy.

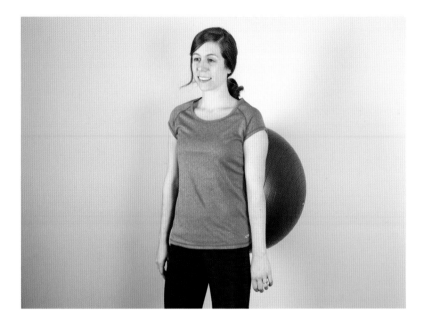

## STEP 1

Stand with back to wall, ball resting against lower back. Feet should be hip distance apart.

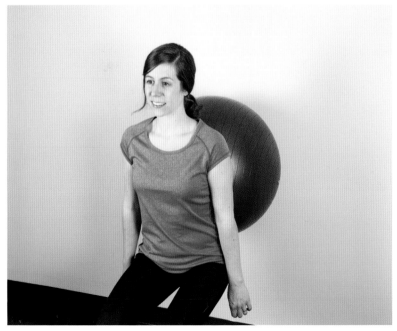

## STEP 2

Keeping upper body straight and abdominals contracted, lower the hips and bend the knees. Be sure that knees are not going past toes.

## STEP 3

Press weight down through the heels to press back up to standing.

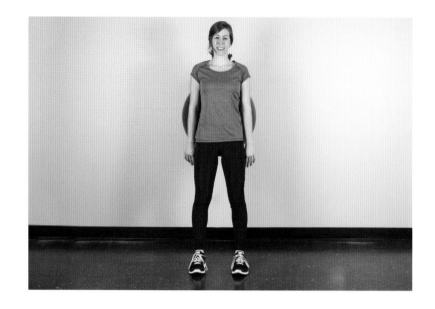

## BRIDGE

This is a low-intensity, no-impact exercise targeting the lower body. The addition of the ball engages the core muscles and aids in balance training. Use caution if suffering from peripheral neuropathy.

## STEP 1

Sit on ball with feet flat on floor.

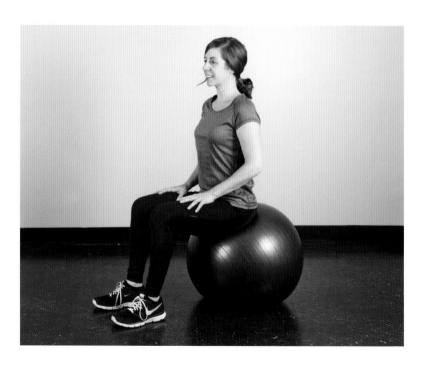

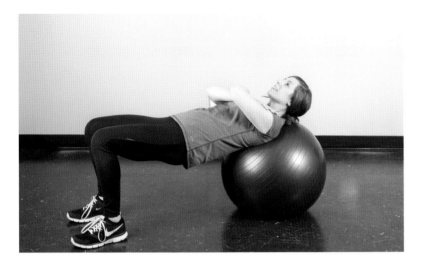

## STEP 2

Walk the feet forward until upper body is resting on the ball, with knees bent at 90 degrees. Cross hands over chest.

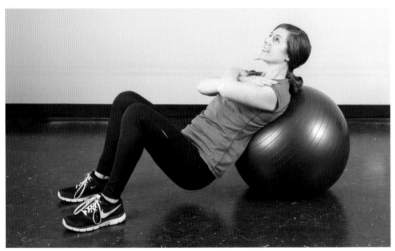

## STEP 3

With tight abdominals, lower the hips until just above the floor.

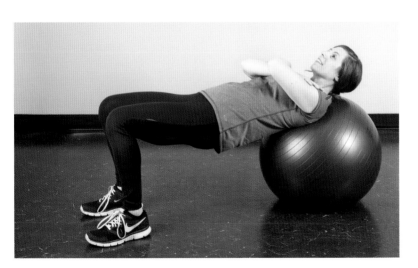

## STEP 4

Keeping abdominals firm, press through the heels to lift the hips back to start position. Do 15 repetitions.

# LIFT AND SQUEEZE

The lift and squeeze is a moderate-intensity, no-impact exercise. This exercise targets the inner thigh muscles that aid in maintaining knee and hip alignment. The core muscles are also challenged while doing this exercise. This exercise is safe for all fitness levels.

## STEP 1

Lie flat on back with feet on either side of stability ball.

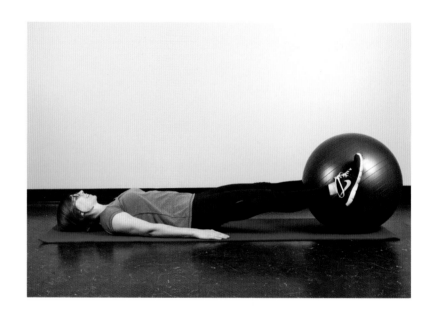

## STEP 2

Squeeze the feet against ball and lift off the ground. Keep lower back pressing into floor or mat, abdominals pulled in.

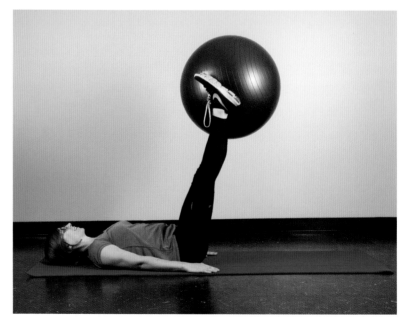

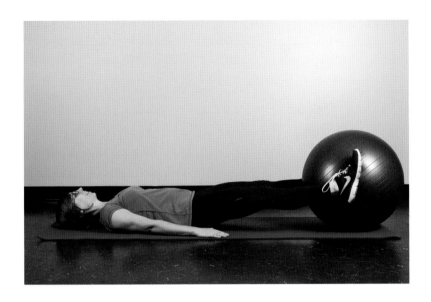

## STEP 3

Keeping the feet squeezed against ball, slowly lower back to ground. Do 10-15 repetitions.

## AB ROLL

This is a moderate-intensity activity targeting the abdominal muscles. Ab rolls can put some strain on the back and knees, so avoid this exercise if any pain occurs.

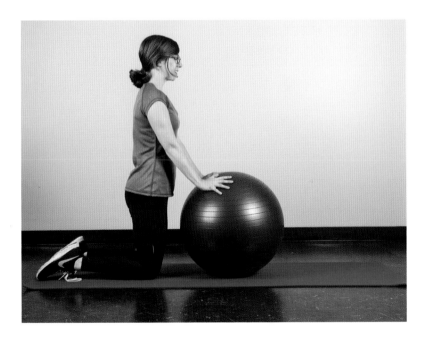

## STEP 1

Kneel on floor in front of ball with hands resting on the ball. Keep your elbows bent and hands parallel.

## STEP 2

Tightening abdominals, roll ball as far forward as comfortable, keeping knees on floor. Keep spine straight. Do not let hips drop.

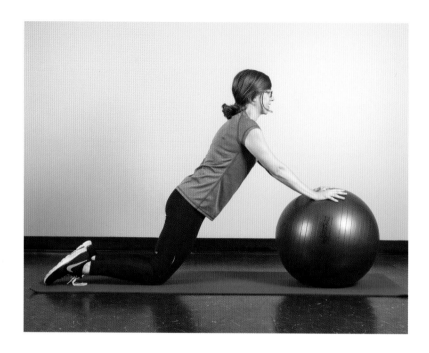

## STEP 3

Pause in rolled out position for one deep breath. Slowly roll back to start. Do 10-15 repetitions.

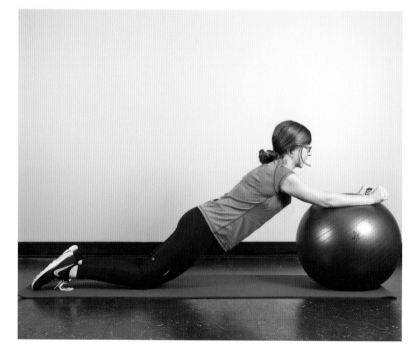

# LEG EXTENSIONS

Leg extensions on a stability ball are a double duty strength and balance exercise; they target the thigh muscles and the core. This low-intensity, no-impact exercise is safe for all fitness levels.

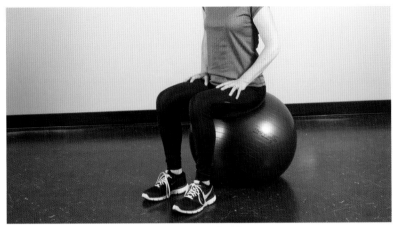

## STEP 1

Sit on ball with feet flat on floor. Place hands on thighs. For more stability, place hands on either side of ball.

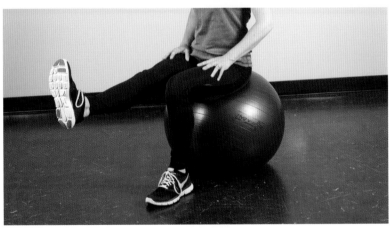

## STEP 2

Sitting tall, lift right leg straight out, toes pointing to ceiling.

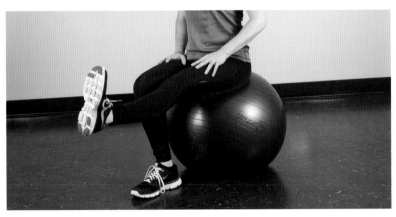

## STEP 3

Lower to start position. Do 10-15 repetitions. Repeat with other leg.

## STEP 4

Lift arms to create a greater balance challenge.

# KNEE LIFTS

Knee lifts on a stability ball target the hip muscles as well as the core and back. This exercise is low intensity and is a double duty exercise that helps not only strength but also balance and posture. This exercise is safe for all fitness levels.

## STEP 1

Sit on ball with feet flat on floor. Place hands on thighs.

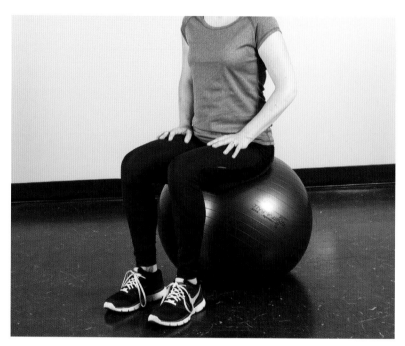

## STEP 2

Sit tall with abdominals tight. Lift knee as high as possible. Do not round forward, but keep a long spine.

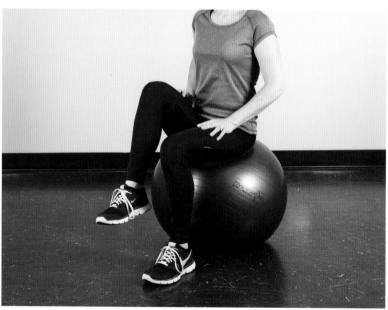

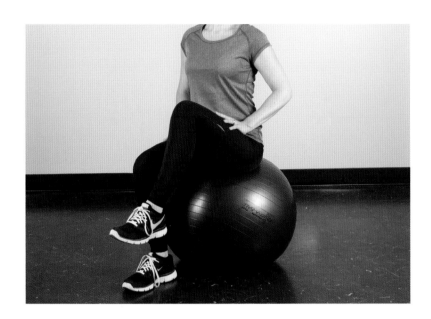

## STEP 3

Lower to start position. Do 10-15 repetitions. Repeat with other leg.

## STEP 4

Lift arms to create a greater balance challenge.

# CALF RAISES

Strong calves are an important element for good balance and proper knee and ankle alignment. Calf raises on the stability ball are a low-intensity, low-impact way to strengthen the calf muscles while also working the core muscles and improving posture. This exercise may not be suitable for people with peripheral neuropathy in the feet.

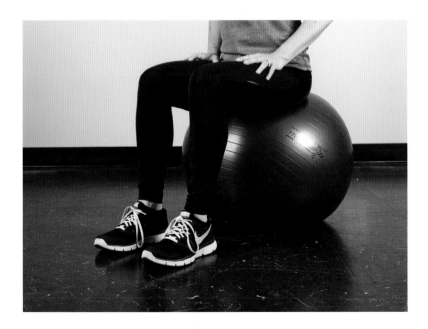

## STEP 1

Sit on the ball with feet at hip distance (feet together for increased balance challenge). Keep spine long and abdominals pulled in.

## STEP 2

Lift left heel off ground, pause. Lower to start position. Do 10–15 repetitions. Repeat with other leg.

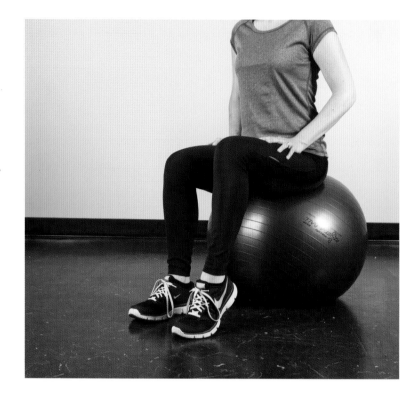

## STEP 3

For added challenge, do both legs.

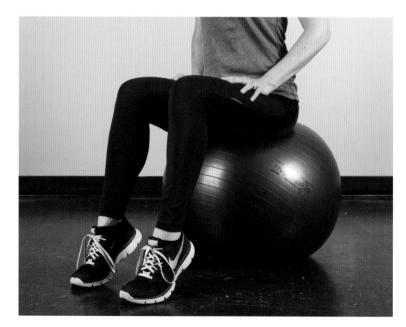

# BICEP CURLS

This is a low-intensity, no-impact exercise. Bicep curls target the muscle on the front of the arm. This muscle is important for lifting and pulling. The addition of the ball helps with core strength and balance. If hand strength is compromised because of neuropathy of the hand, use caution. This exercise can also be done with wrist weights. Do one arm at a time to decrease the challenge, if needed.

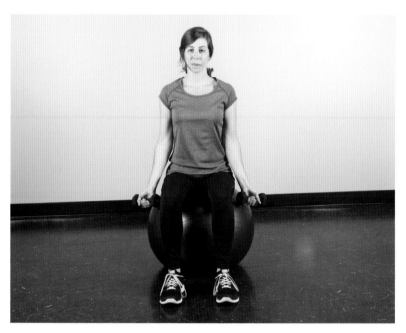

## STEP 1

Sit on ball with feet at hip distance (feet closer together for added balance challenge). Keep spine long and abdominals pulled in. Hold a weight in each hand, palms facing up.

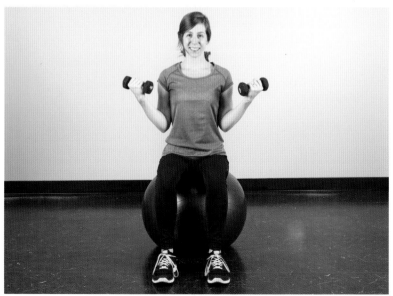

## STEP 2

Keeping elbows close to body, curl hands up toward shoulders, with palms facing up to ceiling. Do 10-15 repetitions.

# CHEST FLY

Chest fly exercises strengthen the muscles in the front of the chest. These muscles are key for good posture. This exercise is a moderate-intensity, no-impact exercise and is safe for all fitness levels. The addition of the ball incorporates core strength and balance.

## STEP 1

Sit on ball, feet at hip distance. Hold a weight in each hand. Walk feet forward until upper back is resting on ball.

## STEP 2

Straighten arms over head so hands are directly over the face, palms in. Arms should be nearly straight, keeping slight bend in elbows.

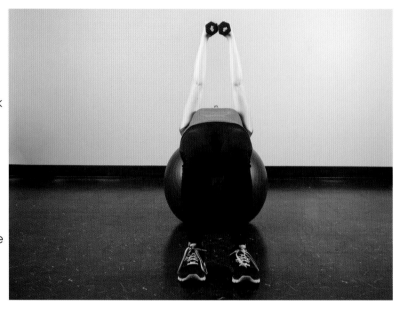

## STEP 3

Lower arms out to sides, keeping elbows slightly bent.

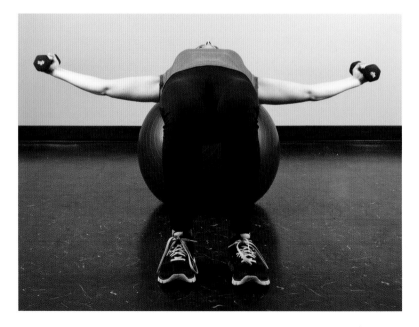

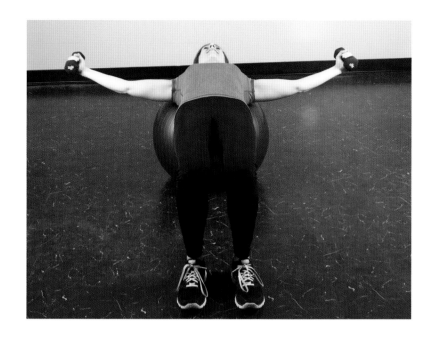

Return to start position. Do 10-15 repetitions.

## TRICEP EXTENSION

This is a low-intensity, no-impact exercise. Tricep extensions work the back of the arms, strengthening the muscles in charge of pulling and pressing. The addition of the ball incorporates core strength and balance.

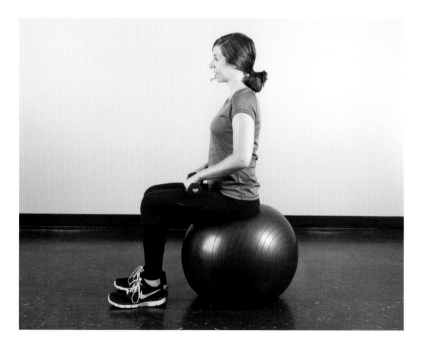

## STEP 1

Sit on ball, feet at hip distance. Hold a weight in each hand.

## STEP 2

Walk feet forward until upper back is resting on ball. Keep hips lifted.

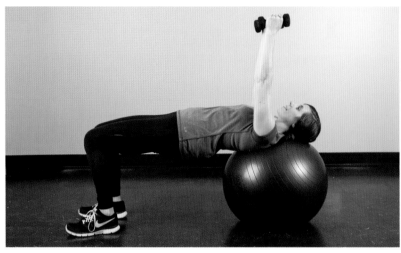

## STEP 3

Straighten arms overhead so hands are directly over the face, palms in. Arms should be straight.

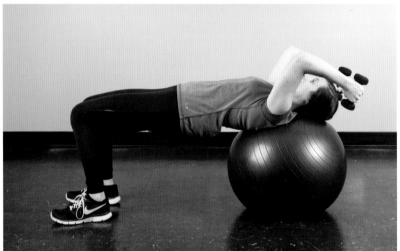

## STEP 4

Bend elbows to 90 degrees, lowering hands behind head.

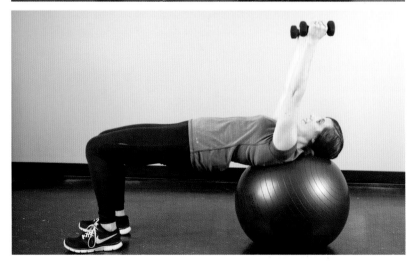

## STEP 5

Press back to start position. Do 10–15 repetitions.

# YOGA POSES

Yoga has become very popular in the last couple of decades, and with good reason. Yoga is a no-impact workout that can be performed at whatever level of intensity is best for you. Higher intensity yoga will burn more calories faster, as many as 500 in an hour-long session, while lower intensity classes burn fewer calories. There are many different kinds of yoga, too, so you can shop around until you find the style that you like best.

Hatha yoga is great for beginners, as it is a very gentle yoga style that emphasizes poses, breathing, and meditation. Bikram yoga, also called "hot" yoga, is also based around postures and breathing, but it is performed in a sauna-like room and can be great for burning lots of calories in a very low-intensity manner. Ashtanga yoga is performed very rapidly and provides an excellent cardio-intensive workout. Restorative yoga uses supportive props like eye pillows and bolsters; it is designed to help alleviate stress and improve relaxation.

Any of these styles will help improve your core strength. As you build abdominal muscle, you'll be able to burn calories faster. And after a good yoga session, you'll feel very relaxed, which will help keep your cortisol levels low.

You can drop in on a yoga class to find out if the instructor and style are right for you. Classes are available at gyms, yoga studios, churches, and community centers. Classes have the advantage that a trained instructor will teach you the different poses and correct your posture, which can be hard to do on your own. Many drop-in classes are very affordable, and some are even free, so you can try out a few different styles before you decide which kind you prefer. Or, if you can't find a class that works with your schedule, you can find instructional yoga DVDs at the library or watch instructional videos online. You can pause the videos and move through the poses at your own pace.

# MOUNTAIN POSE

Mountain Pose is a low-intensity pose that is safe for all fitness levels. This exercise is beneficial for improving posture and lower body strength. It also helps strengthens the core.

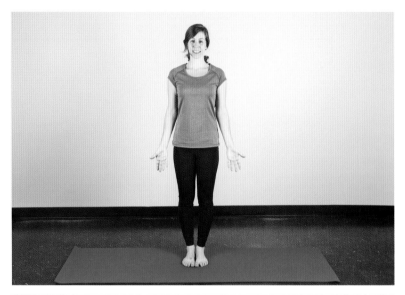

## STEP 1

Stand tall with feet at hip distance. Tuck tailbone in and pull abdominals in toward spine. Relax shoulders; let arms hang by sides with palms facing out.

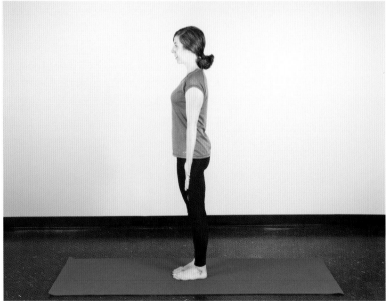

## STEP 2

Reach crown of head toward the ceiling while pushing heels down into floor. Hold for five breaths.

# LOW LUNGE/HIGH LUNGE

Low Lunge is a low-intensity balance pose. This pose may be difficult for people with peripheral neuropathy, so practice with caution. Low Lunge strengthens the lower body as well as relieving pressure caused by sciatica. High Lunge is a moderate-intensity balance pose that aids in stretching the groin and strengthens the legs.

## STEP 1

Begin in Mountain Pose. Step right foot back into a wide leg stance.

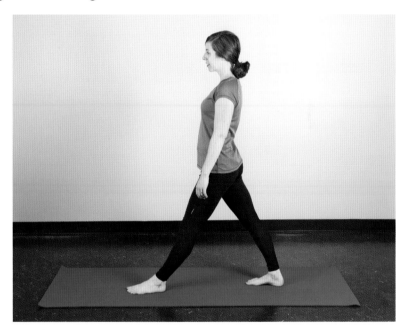

## STEP 2

Bend left knee to 90 degrees while lowering left knee to floor. Straighten left leg as much as possible, pressing hips down toward floor.

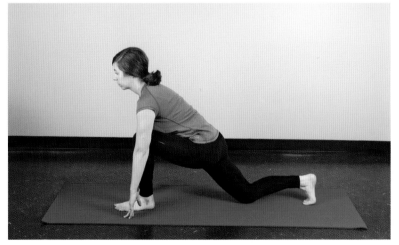

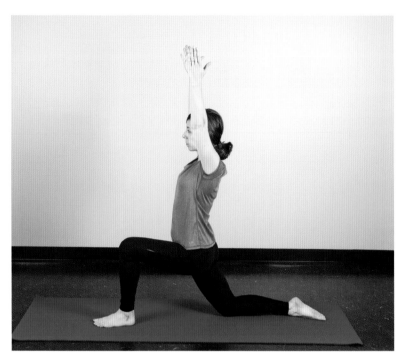

## STEP 3

Place both hands on left knee and straighten upper body. Inhale while sweeping both hands up to the ceiling. For an added balance challenge, look up. Hold for three deep breaths. Repeat with left leg.

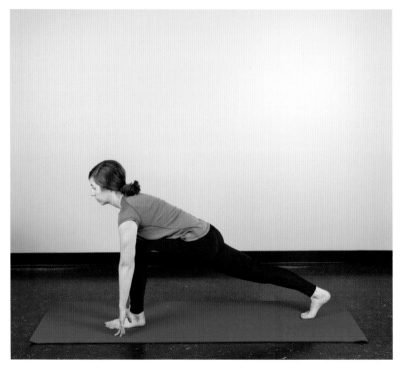

## STEP 4

To move into High Lunge, place fingers on floor for stability and press right leg straight. Repeat steps 2 and 3.

# DOWNWARD FACING DOG

Downward Facing Dog is a moderate-intensity pose. It strengthens and stretches muscles of the entire body and aids in preventing osteoporosis. Benefits include improved digestion and increased energy. Be cautious practicing this pose if carpal tunnel syndrome is present.

## STEP 1

Begin on hands and knees with wrists under shoulders and knees under hips.

## STEP 2

Curling toes under, press hips up to ceiling.

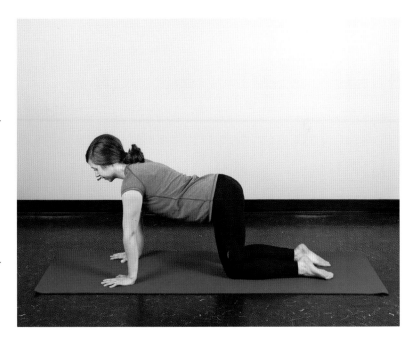

## STEP 3

Adjust body so arms are straight with palms pressing firmly into floor.

## STEP 4

Continue to lift hips up while pressing heels down. Bend knees slightly if pain is felt in legs. Hold for five breaths.

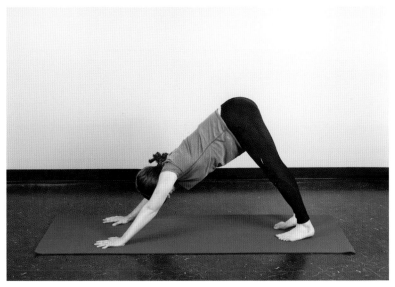

# WARRIOR POSE

Warrior Pose is a moderate-intensity pose designed to strengthen and stretch the legs and ankles. This pose also facilitates core strengthening and balance training. If problems with the neck are present do not turn to look over the fingertips, but keep head forward.

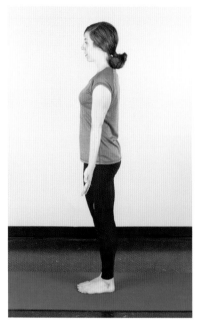 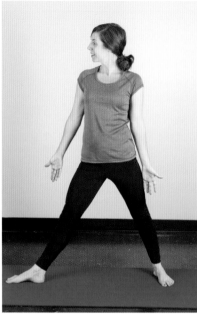

## STEP 1

Begin in Mountain Pose. Step feet about three to four feet apart.

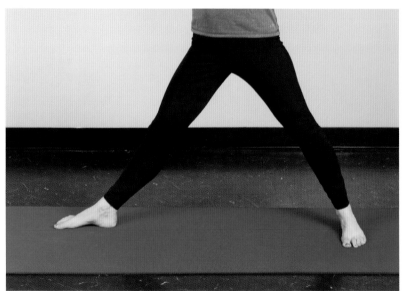

## STEP 2

Turn left foot and knee outward, while right foot remains in place.

## STEP 3

Inhale to sweep arms out to sides. Look over your fingertips.

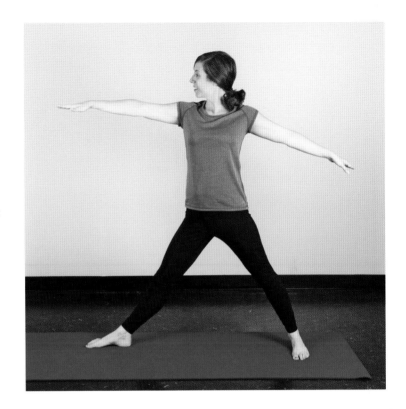

## STEP 4

Bend front leg to 90 degrees. Keep upper body very tall.

## STEP 5

Keeping back leg straight, push outside edge of back foot into floor. Hold for three breaths.

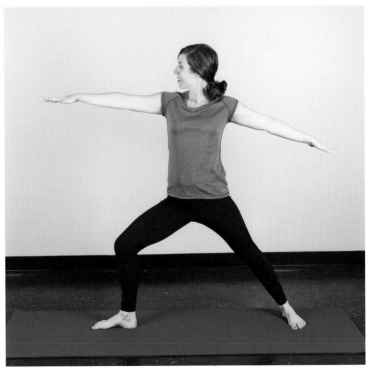

# TREE POSE

This pose is a moderate-intensity balance pose. Tree Pose strengthens the ankles, calves, and thighs. It also promotes strengthening of the core and back. Tree Pose also helps improve focus.

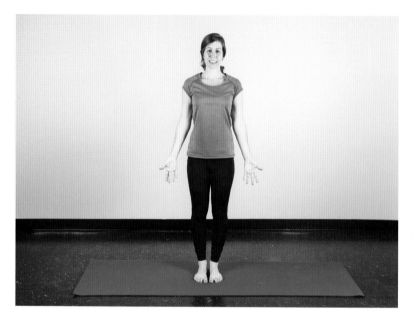

## STEP 1

Begin in Mountain Pose. Rest bottom of right foot against left ankle with knee turned out. If turning knee out causes pain in hip, keep knee pointing forward.

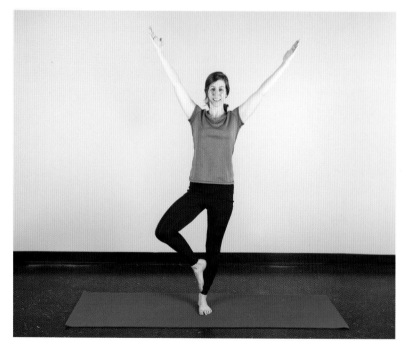

## STEP 2

Keep spine long and abdominals firm. Pull right foot up to shin or thigh. Do not rest foot against knee. Reach both hands up to ceiling. Hold for three deep breaths. Repeat with other leg.

# MOON POSE

Moon pose is a low-intensity pose used to stretch the arms and the sides of the waist.

## STEP 1

Begin in Mountain Pose. Interlace fingers and turn palms down.

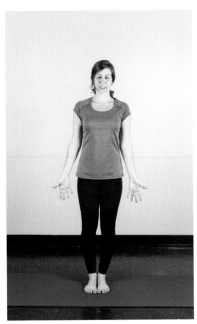 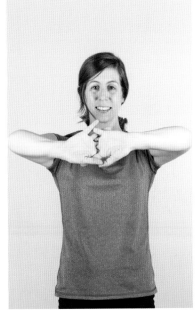

## STEP 2

Inhale hands up over head, palms facing up.

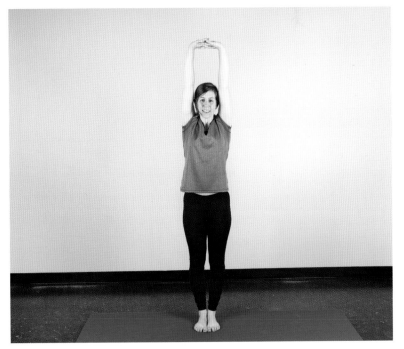

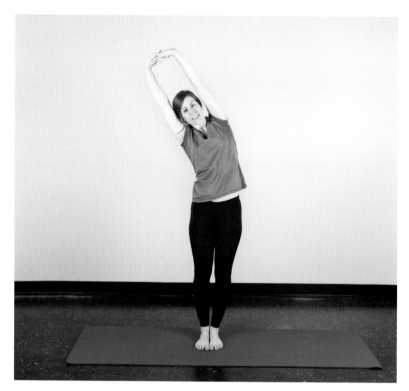

## STEP 3

With hands reaching up, lean upper body to the right. Hold for three deep breaths.

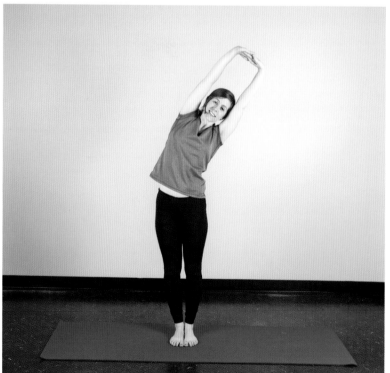

## STEP 4

Repeat on left side.

# CAT/COW

This flow series is low intensity and aids in strengthening and stretching the low back and core muscles. Cat/Cow is a pose used to practice pairing breath with movement, which helps relieve anxiety. Because this pose is done on hands and knees, be cautious if knee or wrist pain occurs.

## ON A MAT

### STEP 1

Begin on hands and knees, with wrists under shoulders and knees under hips.

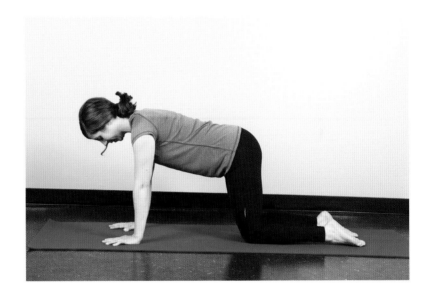

### STEP 2

Inhale while rounding the back.

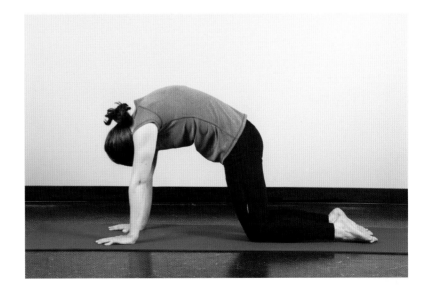

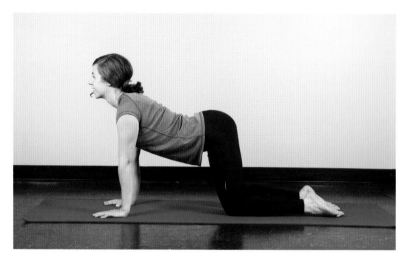

## STEP 3

Exhale while pressing hands and knees into floor, arching back, and looking upward. Each breath pattern equals one set. Continue for five sets.

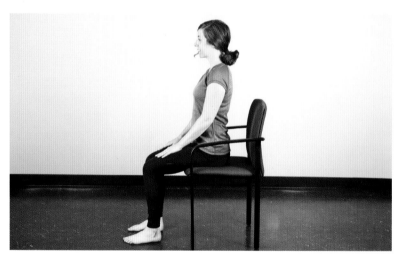

## IN A CHAIR

## STEP 1

Begin seated in chair with hands on thighs.

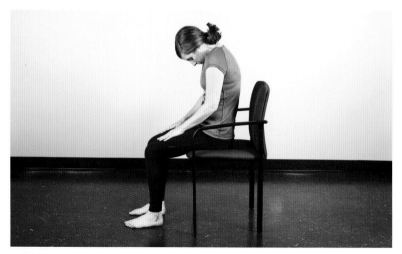

## STEP 2

Inhale while rounding the back.

## STEP 3

Exhale while arching back and looking up to ceiling. Each breath pattern equals one set. Continue for five sets.

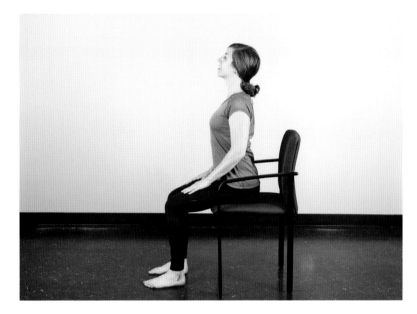

## TRIANGLE POSE

Triangle Pose is a moderate-intensity pose that stretches and strengthens the lower body. It is also helpful in relieving anxiety and stress. If neck pain occurs in this stretch, do not look up at ceiling, but keep head pointing forward.

## STEP 1

Begin in Mountain Pose. Step feet into wide leg stance, about three to four feet apart. Position feet as shown here.

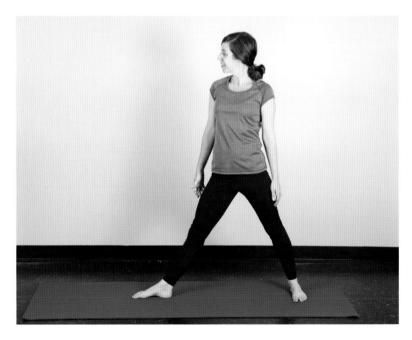

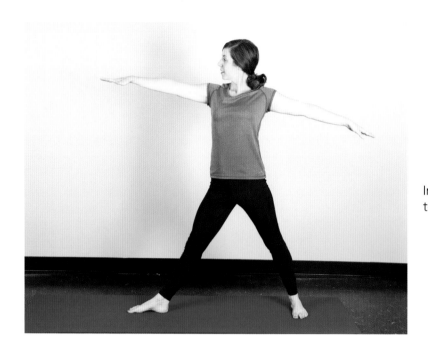

## STEP 2

Inhale arms out
to sides.

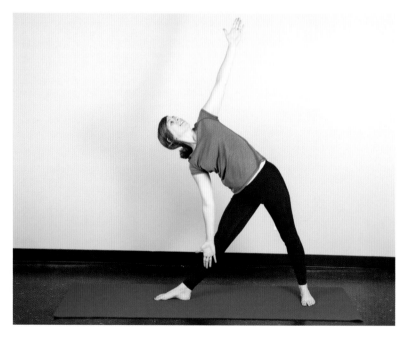

## STEP 3

Exhale to reach right
hand to shin or ankle.
Left arm reaches up
to the ceiling. If it's
comfortable, turn the
head to look up at
left arm. Keep back
straight, tailbone
tucked under.

## STEP 4

Hold for three deep breaths, then repeat on other side.

## BOUND ANGEL POSE

This pose is a low-intensity pose that promotes stimulation of the heart and improves circulation. Other benefits include decreased stress, anxiety, and depression. Bound Angel Pose focuses on stretching the inner thigh, groin, and knees. If hip, groin, or knee pain is present, sit up on a pillow or yoga block.

## STEP 1

Sit tall with feet flat on floor, knees bent.

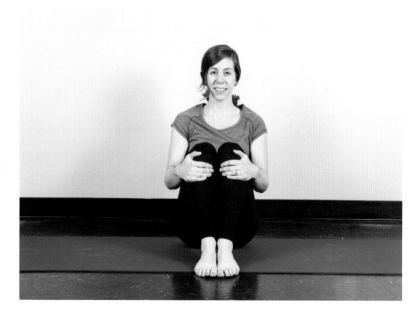

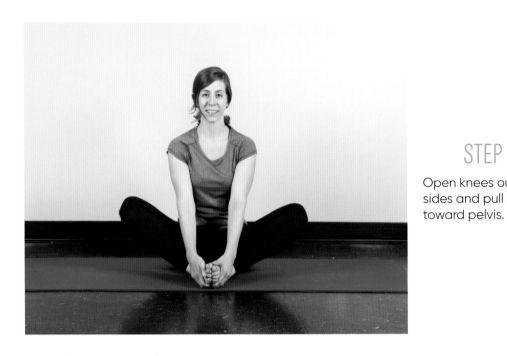

## STEP 2

Open knees out to sides and pull heels in toward pelvis.

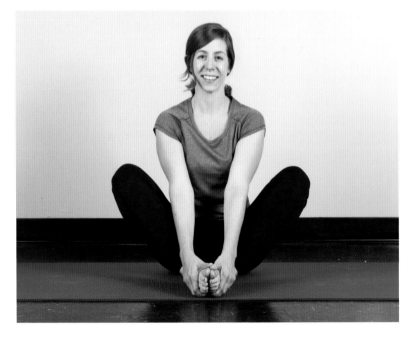

## STEP 3

Place hands around feet.

## STEP 4

Round forward, bringing head towards feet. Hold for three deep breaths.

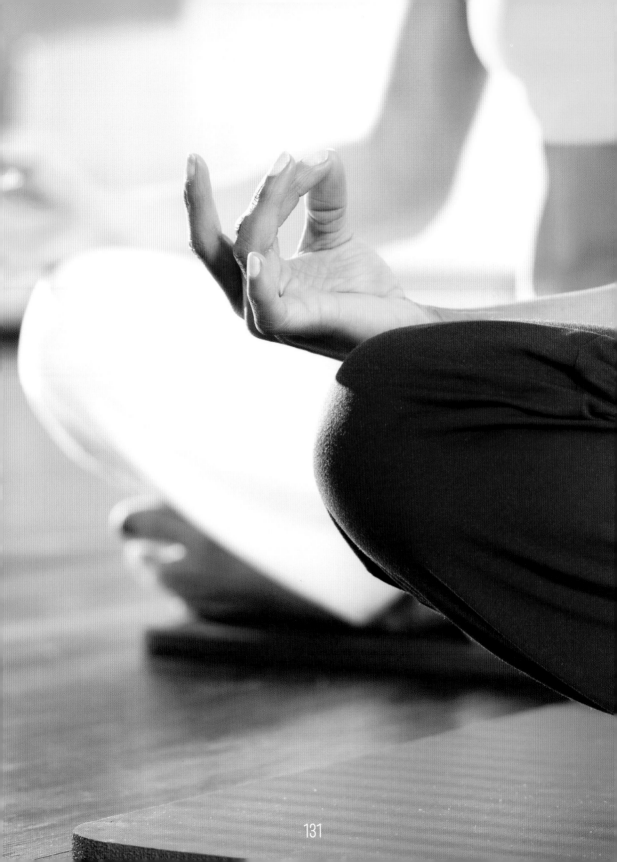

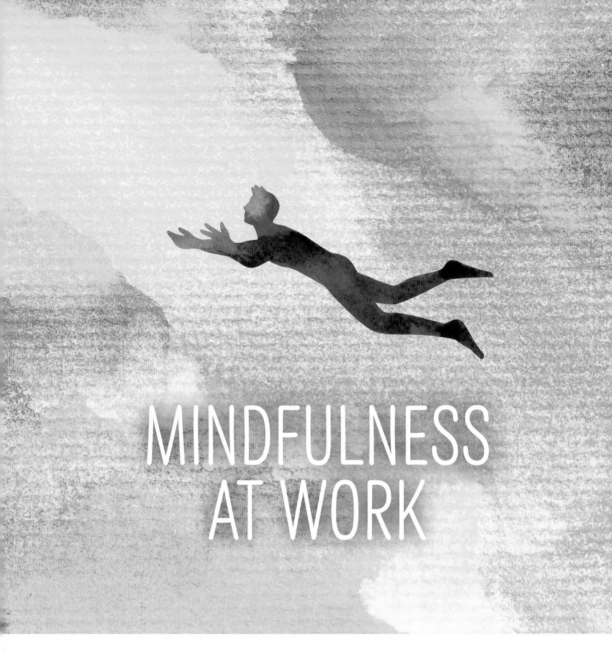

# MINDFULNESS
# AT WORK

Bringing mindfulness into the busy, chaotic workplace may sound impossible, but nowhere is it more needed. Whether you work at home, part-time, full-time, in a small office or a huge corporation, there are workplace stresses that arise from the moment you clock in until the moment you go home. Often, you are required to take your work home with you. That means less time to unwind from the daily grind with family or alone in a warm bath with a fun television show or a good book.

Work has become synonymous with who you are. "What do you do for a living?" is often asked even before someone knows your full name and where you live. Work defines you and even becomes the focal point of your life.

A Gallup poll found that people in the United States work an average of 34.5 hours a week, with full-time workers averaging 47 hours. Self-employed business owners work about 80 hours a week, which is much higher than any other nation in the world. That is a lot of time to spend tense, stressed out, worried about what happened at last week's meeting, or panicked over next month's presentation.

How can you possibly achieve a state of mindfulness in the midst of your busy day, especially when your coworkers are getting on your last nerves and your boss is demanding more work in less time? Is it possible to find time to practice mindfulness when the copier is broken, the delivery person is late, and the bank lost your company deposit? You can, and you must!

Mindfulness in the workplace is a wonderful way to increase focus, make better decisions, increase energy and productivity, and bring colleagues and coworkers into alignment with a shared goal of

raising the company's performance. Mindfulness practice can be solo, but including your coworkers makes the workplace run more efficiently.

Studies show that more people die of heart attacks on Monday mornings than any other time of the week. They dread going to work and repeating the same tasks in the same setting over and over again. By bringing a mindfulness practice into work, you can change your attitude and feelings toward your job, boss, coworkers, commute, and anything else associated with your working world.

Becoming mindful in the workplace doesn't require running off into a

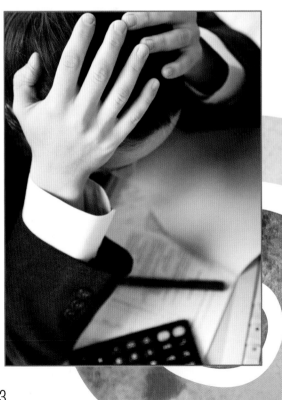

supply closet to do a 30-minute meditation or yoga positions; however, if that is a possibility, it's a great way to spend part of your lunch hour. Mindfulness can be achieved at your desk, in your car as you park before going into the office, in an elevator going up to your office floor, or even in the middle of an important meeting.

## WORKING MEDITATION

Though you cannot actually spend your whole workday meditating, you can spend it in a grounded, centered, and aware state. The conscious effort of entering your workspace with the intention of staying as much in the present moment as possible can go a long way when you start to get caught up in the emails, phone calls, and in-person demands. Taking a few deep breaths as you sit down at your desk, or go to your workstation, can help set you up for the start of your day.

As the day goes by, it's important to stay connected to the present, and you can do that by taking little "check-ins" and noticing the sights, sounds, and smells around you (even the annoying ones). Engaging the senses is a wonderful way to bring your mind back to the present and not dwell in the past or fantasize

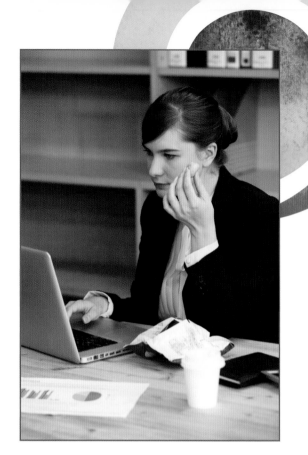

about the future while on the job. Your productivity will soar, and your energy will stay high without caffeine and sugary carbs.

Providing full attention to whatever arises in the course of the day keeps you present and in the moment, even if all you are doing is reading emails or having lunch in the break room. Say, "I am here" if you need to bring the mind's inner narrator back into focus.

# MINI-MEDITATION BREAKS

Take advantage of breaks to regroup with some quick breathing exercises, rather than heading straight for the personal messages and social networking. There will be plenty of time for that when you get home, but while on the job, it's important to use the time you have for refilling the well of ideas, energy, and motivation you may have lost while dealing with your workload.

Washing your hands in the bathroom or break room is a chance to tune in to the sensation of water against your skin. Is it warm? Cold? Is the soap scented? What does it smell like? Are the paper towels soft or do they feel like sandpaper? These may seem like silly questions, but how often do you really notice what you're doing and feeling unless it's some overwhelming experience? Peace and calm can be found in the little things, too. The smaller chores and tasks, even copying something at the copy machine or stapling reports together, are opportunities to strengthen your ability to stay present and be aware of your surroundings.

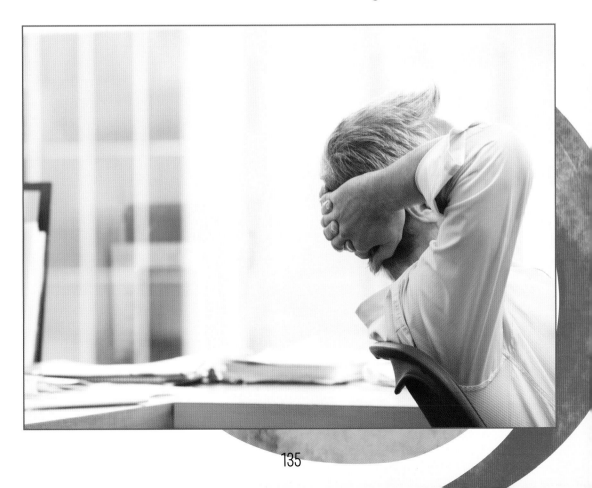

With the many meditation apps available, a five-minute breather can become a refreshing and rejuvenating mini-meditation to finish the rest of your workday on a high note. If you don't have your cell phone nearby, you can plug mini-meditations and mindfulness breaks into your personal calendar or desk calendar or pick a visual "mantra" image and put a picture of it where you can see it as a reminder to take a breather. You can let your coworkers and boss know what you are doing so they too can try it.

## TAKE IT A TASK AT A TIME

Often you must multitask to get things done, but don't be fooled by the "more you do, the faster it all gets done" theory. By focusing on one issue at a time, you open your mind to the present moment power of solutions, choices, and options you may not have had before because you were juggling responsibilities. You give your best, not just a percentage of it, because where focus goes, energy flows. Multitasking or working in a state of worry and anxiety often leads to mistakes and inaccuracies that can come back to haunt you.

One day at a time, one hour at a time, one moment at a time, one task at a time. Mindfulness means being wholly present to whatever you are doing right now. Keeping a priority list can help you identify what task you want to focus on first. You don't want to end up spending so much time grabbing for the low-hanging fruit that you forget to address the bigger, tastier fruit at the top. You might want to answer all pertinent emails in the first hour, go through paperwork in the next hour, and then schedule any meetings for later in the day. Blocking time like this can keep you organized, freeing your focus and attention to really examine what you

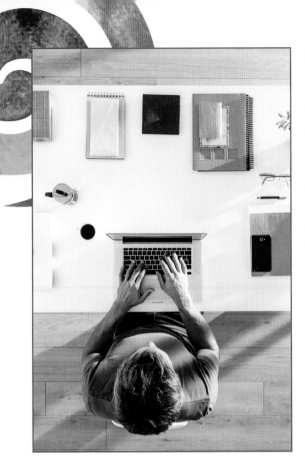

computer, make sure your desktop isn't cluttered with a hundred folders and documents that overwhelm your brain every time you look at them. Keep general folders marked by project name, and put everything pertinent to that project in the folder. You can leave the top priority item on your desktop to work on, then put that in the folder when finished and move your next priority project to the desktop. "First things first" goes a long way to getting the most important items done first, leaving the rest of your day to deal with less critical tasks when your energy level might be lower.

Using a calming desktop screensaver can be a lovely reminder to breathe. Visuals are powerful aids for staying in the moment, so make the image something that soothes you every time you look at it. It might even be a motivational quote or saying, like "Go for your dreams," or "Live in the moment." Set your screensaver to come on only when your desktop is idle so as not to distract you from the project you are working on. You can adjust timing in your settings to fit your needs.

are doing and make sure you are doing it well.

Where do you work? In an office? A cubicle? A desk out in the middle of a busy warehouse? No matter where you call your workspace home, you can keep it a haven for mindfulness. Start by decluttering your space, especially your desk. It's impossible to keep your focus in the present moment when there are 10 stacks of pending work folders on your desk. A clean, organized desk makes for a clear, organized mind.

If you keep your work files on a

Keeping something on your desk such as a beloved object or photograph serves the same purpose. Even fresh flowers can bring you back into the moment

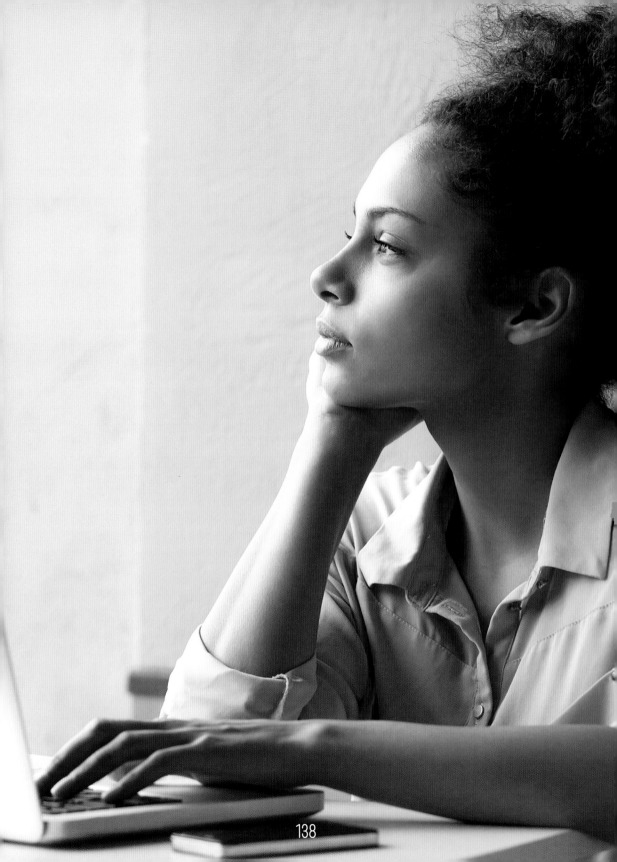

during a stressful day. Stopping to smell the roses, or whatever flower of your choice, reminds you of the beauty of the present and the value of slowing down. Maybe you choose a photo of your spouse or your children. Maybe you find a gorgeous postcard of a vacation spot you hope to visit soon. Whatever is important and meaningful to you, find a place for it on your desk. It should calm you, soothe you, and even bring a smile to your face.

## ATTITUDE ADJUSTMENTS

Being at work often provokes feelings of anxiety, resentment, and even anger. If you don't like your boss—or worse, your job—you might find yourself depressed the whole time you are on the job. That's a lot of hours spent feeling miserable, so perhaps a great mindfulness exercise involves an adjustment of your attitude to help bring you back to your center. Think about how much time you spend at work wishing you were home. Or how often your mind drifts to the time spent last weekend or three months from now when you'll be on vacation. Before you know it, eight hours have passed, and along with them, the gifts of the present moment they offered.

Several times a day, stop and engage with your feelings. Angry? Rushed? Chaotic? Bored to tears? Ask yourself what you can be grateful for right now, in that very job with that very boss and those very colleagues. Are you grateful to have a job in the first place? Do you like the fact that your workplace is so close to your home that you have a short commute? Does your boss have a good sense of humor? Do you have colleagues you actually go out with outside of work and enjoy being in their company? Do you get free business cards on the job?

Entering a state of gratitude helps you find reasons to feel better about the circumstances you are currently in, regardless of your intention to stay at that job or not. An attitude of gratitude demands you be in the present, looking at your blessings with open and alert eyes, and being aware of the good things alongside the bad. There are always good things if you seek them.

## SERENITY NOW!

Job sites can be noisy and busy, so much so that finding a moment of peace is all but impossible. Yet every work situation offers the chance to find a moment or two of serenity, even if you have to dash outside or put on a pair of headphones to block out the distractions. Some

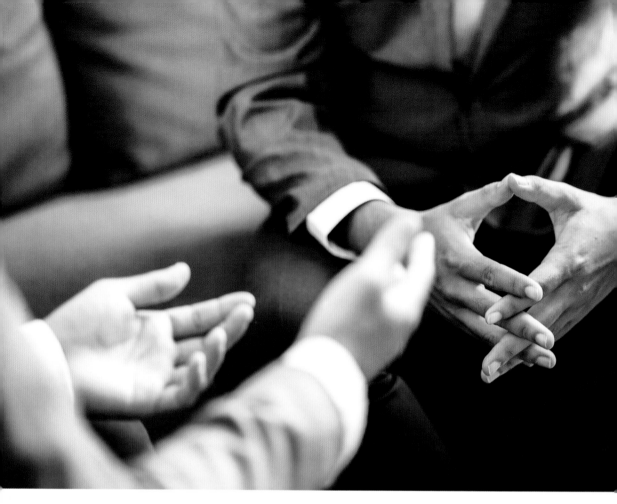

people thrive on chaos, but even they need a break to keep their energy and productivity high.

Don't be afraid to seek out opportunities to sneak some serenity into your day. If you have an office, close the door for 10 minutes and put out a DO NOT DISTURB sign. Nothing is so important it cannot wait 10 minutes, and in most cases, your peace of mind is more important than any interruption.

## ENGAGE!

You work with other people, but how often do you really engage with them? Mindfulness includes being there with others in a way that makes them feel the full force of your attention. Put down the cell phone and close the email when you are in a meeting or need to address an issue with a coworker. Give them the gift of your interested presence and, if needed, your appreciation and compassion.

This is critical with challenging coworkers and bosses. Sitting down and listening to one another rather than brushing disagreements under the rug can alleviate office tension. You often spend more time with these people than your own family, after all. When you are all in sync, you all benefit from increased productivity and improved morale.

Perhaps people are on their cell phones during conference calls and meetings. You can practice mindfulness by putting your phone away and totally immersing yourself in the call or meeting subject matter. This is your job, and you have an investment in the company you

work for, so why would you not want to be engaged in the ups and downs of how that company is run? Being present often brings a new appreciation for your job when you become aware of the infrastructure and inner workings of the company.

If you work alone, you may take virtual meetings and conference calls. The same rule should apply. Put the phone away and stop multitasking to engage with your clients, customers, and colleagues. When you give them your full attention, they will reciprocate, creating a stronger relationship that benefits both sides. People know when you are not fully paying attention to them and will often hold back from offering their best solutions and ideas. They will match your energy at the level you offer it, so be present and give them your best to get their best in return.

## BRINGING MINDFULNESS INTO THE WORKPLACE

More and more corporations and institutions like Google and Harvard Business School are finding ways to bring mindfulness into the workplace, even training their workers and offering leadership programs to teach mindfulness principles that can increase efficiency and communications

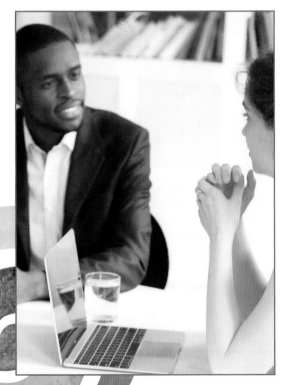

and reduce stress and conflict. Mindfulness programs can teach workers to prioritize time, brainstorm ideas and solutions, feel more refreshed, and even bring those positive benefits home with them at the end of the workday.

Because mindfulness is associated with increased emotional intelligence, self-regulation, and empathy, it makes sense that it is being considered in more companies as a valid part of employee instruction. Just as you might take a course in how to use the company's computer system, you can learn how to be a better colleague and communicate your needs better via a mindfulness study on the job. If your company doesn't have one, suggest one and take the initiative to tell your supervisors the benefits of incorporating mindfulness practices like short meditation breaks or longer lunch periods.

You might even suggest some mindfulness seminars or group games that can be played in the conference room to sharpen focus

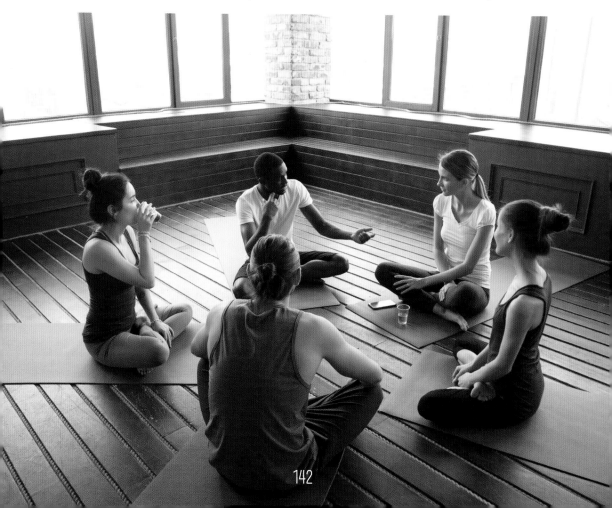

and awareness, including ways to find solutions to a problem by using in-the-moment thinking and strategizing. No cell phones or distractions are allowed. You can even look into having a professional come and teach your office the skills needed to improve working conditions. Many companies allow employees to attend career advancement seminars, so why not create a one-day seminar or one-hour class that teaches you to be more peaceful, present, and productive?

## CONFLICT RESOLUTION

Mindfulness at work is easy when the days go well. But what happens when there is major conflict and tension? The boss is upset about something that happened and takes it out on you. Your colleague takes credit for a huge project you did all the work on. The phone system goes down, the copier is on the fritz, and the building is on lockdown. If something can go wrong, it will. Staying mindful goes a long way to resolving big and small challenges by keeping you focused on the exact nature of the problem so that you can keep your cool and seek solutions in even the craziest of situations.

Think of a fire in the building. Does

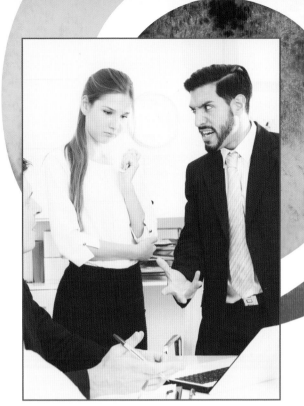

dwelling on the past or being anxious about the future help you find your way out to safety? No, but being totally alert and focused on the fire evacuation plan your office has in place does. Conflicts, emergencies, disasters, and fights are difficult enough to deal with, but if you keep your eyes on what you need to do right now, at that moment, the outcome will be a whole lot more satisfying, and in the case of an actual disaster, can save your life.

As a boss or manager, being mindful and giving your total awareness to your employees makes them feel heard and respected. Conflicts or

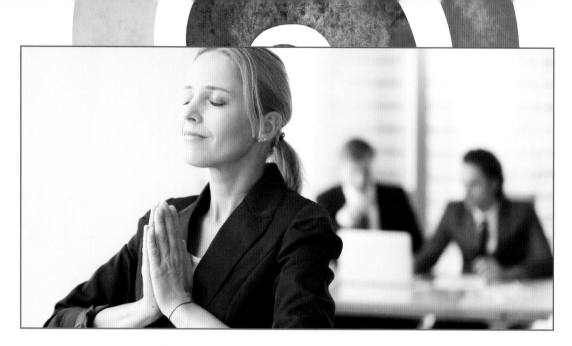

resentments are easily overcome when you show your employees that you are fully listening to their complaints and issues. No one likes to work for a hassled and stressed boss who yells and throws things. A calm boss reflects on his or her employees, making them feel more involved, comfortable, and appreciated.

As an employee, mindfulness increases your ability to function at a high level. If you are looking for a promotion or a raise, the outcome is better served when you have a track record of being on the ball and sharp, present, and engaged in the company. Managers would much rather have employees who are ready to accept challenges than those who complain and waste time with distractions.

Other people are out of your control, but you can control your reactions and responses to them. When a workplace battle emerges, you can stay present and not be swayed by emotions. Conflicts often occur when there is a breakdown of communication; people no longer "hear" each other over their own thoughts and needs. Mindfulness keeps everyone open and present so they can all be heard, acknowledged, and considered when finding a solution.

## COMMUTING

Many people are forced to commute to work, often sitting in traffic for hours both ways, or they are stuck on overcrowded mass transportation systems. Just the act of getting to work and back home is taxing to the spirit and exhausting to the mind and body. Practicing mindfulness while commuting can turn those hours into something beneficial. If you are stuck in traffic, use that time to deep breathe. You may choose to just stay present to the flow of traffic, the cars around you, and the people in those cars. Offer a smile when your car pulls up alongside another. Wave someone in as they try to merge. Mindfulness can include small acts of kindness.

Riding public transportation is a wonderful time to perform a short mindfulness meditation. Look around at the people you are riding with. Without staring, imagine what their lives might be like, and wish them well in your mind, if not out loud, as they disembark at their stations or stops. Look out the window and take in the scenery. You may see things about your city you never noticed before, like a new restaurant or a park you can visit on the weekends.

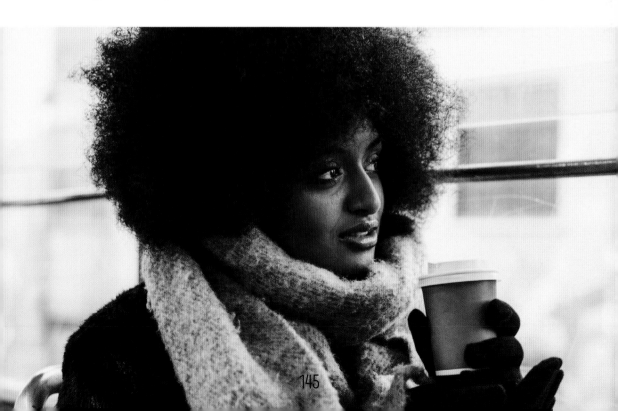

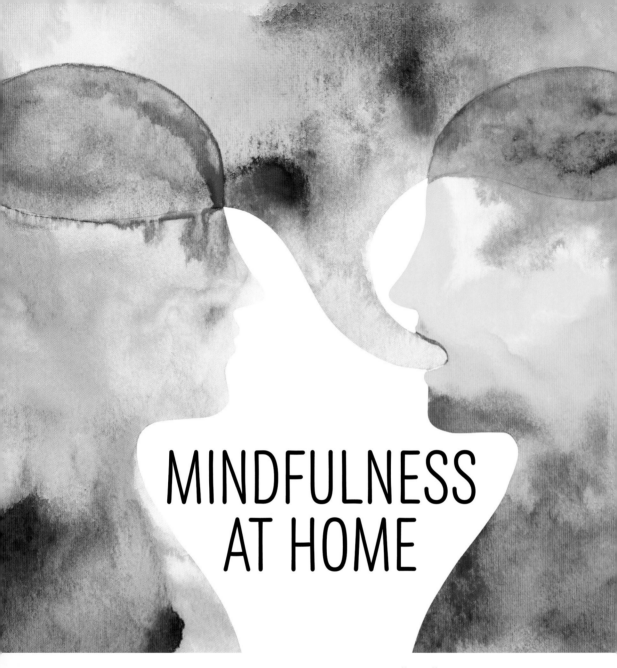

# MINDFULNESS AT HOME

Happiness begins at home, so the saying goes. But with all of life's demands, inner peace and well-being may be elusive and challenging. There are the demands of spouses, children, aging parents, home maintenance and repairs, pets, and bills, all intruding on your ability to stay present. Even with the most dedicated mindfulness practice, there will be times when the home front will feel more like a war zone instead of the safe haven and happy retreat it's supposed to be.

Allowing mindfulness to become a part of the everyday routine involves commitment, especially when children are involved. But the benefits of keeping home a place where everyone looks forward to spending time after work or school are tremendous. Without this sanctuary, you may feel as though you can never truly relax, recharge, and regroup.

Including time for mindfulness practice is critical; there is always something else we could do with that time. Excuses are abundant, so make it as fixed on your calendar as a doctor's visit or a dinner party with friends. You will be far more likely to stick to it if you plan it into each day, week, and month. Eventually, the goal is to be mindful and live in the present without having to think about it too much. It becomes a new habit.

People on their deathbeds rarely wish they'd had more time to worry, stress out over the future, or work more. Rather, they wish they had had more time with family, children, and friends. They wish they had been mindful of time passing.

Even if you live alone (or with furry pet roommates), mindfulness helps you cope with the pressures that come with creating and maintaining a nurturing and comfortable space to call your own. Making your home a retreat starts with clearing out what is no longer needed or used.

## SACRED SPACE

You will never feel clear in a cluttered space. Mindfulness begins with a clear mind, but how can you achieve that when your living space is cramped and crowded, filled with stuff you either don't like or don't need? You can't help but notice the accumulating dust, the piles of things to be sorted through, the way the storage space in your garage is getting smaller and smaller. Clutter clutters everything. It closes in on you and makes you feel restricted.

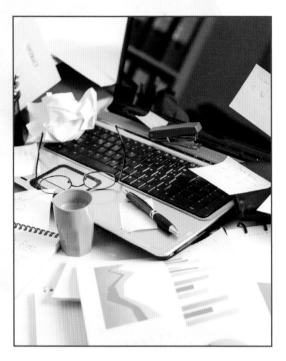

clear out the unnecessary, it's amazing how much better you feel with the newfound space you've created, mentally and physically, and the knowledge that what you no longer use can now be useful to someone else.

Making your home a beautiful place that reflects you or your family's values and personalities is paramount to mindfulness. When your home is peaceful, comfy, and inviting, your home becomes a place to look forward to spending time in rather than a prison to get away from.

Start a home mindfulness practice by gathering your loved ones (or yourself if you live alone) and tidying up each room, putting items in their rightful places, and making a charity pile of anything you don't want or need. This can include books, kitchen gadgets, clothing, toys, furniture, and knickknacks that are taking up space and collecting dust.

You can even have a garage sale and make some money with items you no longer use. If you have belongings in the garage piling up to the ceiling or stuck in an off-site storage room that costs you money every month, you'll always feel antsy and anxious. You may not connect those feelings to being surrounded by too much clutter. Yet once you

The most important rooms for mindfulness practice are bedrooms. Find a spot in your bedroom where you can set up a meditation area with a yoga mat or floor pillow and some scented candles. Create a sign to put on the bedroom door during morning and evening meditations so a spouse looking for the spatula or a child who needs help for a math quiz does not interrupt you.

Encourage children to keep their rooms clear of clutter and to find a special place for their own relaxation and meditation practice. This makes them feel responsible and mature and allows them to have their own little haven to retreat to after a long day of school.

# CONNECTION PROTECTION

Many people are turning their homes into no-gadget zones. When parents get home from work, they turn off cell phones and stay off tablets and gadgets to encourage time to talk with each other and with their children. Getting children to get off their gadgets is quite a tall order, but implementing a no-gadget zone during dinnertime is a good start. How sad is it to see a family sitting around the dinner table, noses buried in their cell phones? This is a time to talk, laugh, listen, and share.

Children who grow up with distracted parents suffer lower self-esteem and lack strong self-acceptance. They feel unheard and unacknowledged. This applies to marriages, too, if spouses are always more concerned with what movie they can watch on a streaming service or who is posting what on social networking sites. There is always time for that later, but society has allowed "tech time" to take precedence over "human time," and everyone is suffering as a result. Isolation, loneliness, anxiety, and depression—these are at an all-time

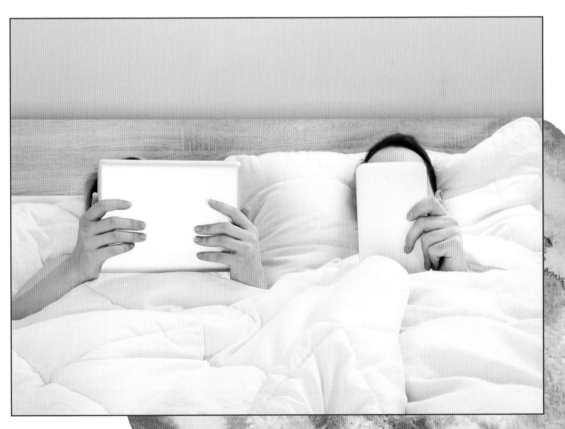

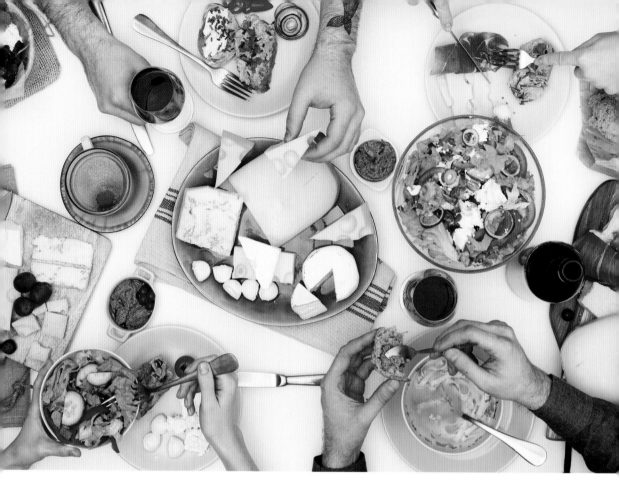

high despite the newfound ability to connect with others all over the world in less than a minute. Humans miss vital face-to-face connection and interaction. Such connections begin in the home.

Dinnertime can become a collective mindfulness game. Go around the table and check in with each family member. Let them talk about their day, the good and the bad. Actively listen and, when the person is done talking, offer support or advice if they ask for it. Too often people focus not on what others are saying but on their own responses. This keeps the mind future-focused, and you lose out on the opportunity of a deeper connection with the person talking to you. Listen. Then respond. Stay present. Don't anticipate your responses. Above all, be mindful of the people you share your table, and your home, with. You may learn things about them that you never knew before!

There must be time for spouses to connect with each other, too. Hire a babysitter or drop the kids off with a family member and have a date night. No talking about past messes or future stresses. The focus is on one another enjoying each other's company.

Date nights or day trips together can bring back that wonderful feeling of curiosity, awe, and wonder as you discover each other all over again and reignite the love that got buried under jobs, bills, and dirty diapers.

Parents can teach their children a valuable lesson in human connection by making bedtime a time for sitting with each child and allowing the child to talk about his or her private concerns away from siblings. Tucking a child in to sleep is a great opportunity to remind your child how loved and appreciated they are. Too often you rush to get your kids to sleep so you can go sit on the couch and unwind, but one day they will be grown and no longer need that "mommy" or "daddy" time, and you will miss it dearly.

Take advantage of being present with your children any chance you can get. You will not regret it.

## FAMILY MEETINGS

Many families impose a weekly family meeting during which everyone airs their grievances and offer suggestions on how to solve family problems affecting everyone involved. These meetings can occur whenever they are needed, especially when conflict arises or when a big decision must be made. But having a regular "check-in time" allows everyone the opportunity to look forward to having the full attention of their fellow family members, even if there is nothing important to discuss.

These meetings are not times for phones, television, reading mail, or opening packages. They are times for sitting around the table and being totally and completely present with one another. In roundabout style, each family member gets the "floor" to talk about whatever they want, without being judged or interrupted. The other members respectfully listen. They will have their own turn to have the floor. Too often, family members complain they are not heard or understood by their loved ones when the problem is they aren't taking the time to be heard or understood.

Just as family meetings offer a chance to fix a problem, family outings offer a time for getting out of the house together and going on a vacation or day trip. Gadgets either stay at home or are only permitted in an emergency. The whole family can have fun deciding where the next family outing will be. The idea is to venture out into the world as a unit and enjoy the day or week together without distractions or interruptions and incorporate conversations over meals, group activities, and quiet downtime.

## PRESSING THE PAUSE BUTTON

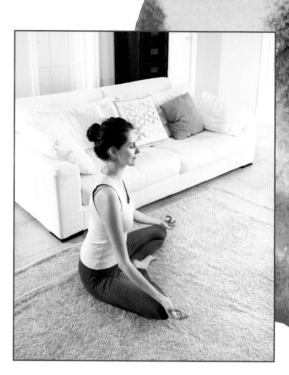

Pressing the pause button on life is a wonderful technique you can employ when things are getting too overwhelming. Imagine having a giant red PAUSE button in your brain. Whenever you feel like you're off balance, exhausted, annoyed, or on the verge of losing your mind, you press the button, stop whatever you are doing, and practice mindfulness. That can be five to 10 deep belly breaths, a five-minute meditation, or a bubble bath. You forget, during the pause, about whatever you were worrying about, knowing you can always return attention to it later if needed.

Once you pause you often find the problem wasn't as big or as intimidating as you first thought, and the solutions come without force or effort. A pause is perfect anywhere, but at home it can mean the difference between yelling at your spouse or child or taking a step back and becoming present.

Teach your children to imagine their own inner pause button they can press when life at home or even at school gets to be too much. When fear, anxiety, or worry presents itself, your child can press the pause button, breathe, close his or her eyes, and relax. Children can utilize their inner pause button when they have too much homework to do and feel overwhelmed. You can even make them an actual big red button with the word PAUSE on it for their bedrooms.

## CHILDREN AND MINDFULNESS

Children can usually learn to meditate and achieve a state of mindfulness much easier than adults.

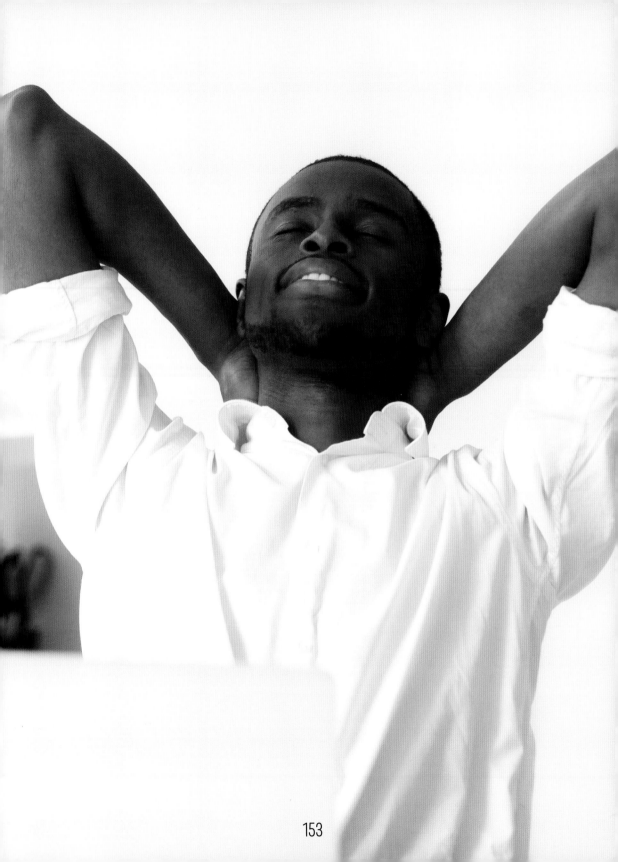

Young children exist in the present, for the most part. Only later when they enter school and experience the pressures of growing up do they start to fret over the past and worry about the future, taking them out of those wonderful times of just being alive in the moment. Cultivating their ability to stay present is a high priority and a tool that will help them solve problems and find solutions in all areas of life. Mindfulness keeps the awe and wonder of childhood alive even as they become teenagers and ultimately adults.

There are books, audiotapes, computer programs, and phone apps geared toward teaching children mindfulness techniques. Start out by talking about mindfulness with your children and showing them the various techniques. Then, let them do experimenting on their own to discover what works for them. Some children love gadgets, so download meditation apps. Other children love to read, and there is no shortage of reading material in book form or online. Once they are properly instructed on the basics, let them create their own mindfulness practice. Keep a chart of their progress on the refrigerator or bedroom wall and reward them with a fun treat.

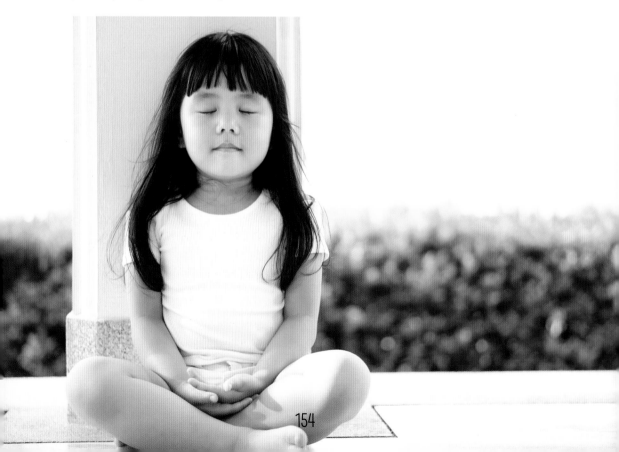

Children experience constant anxieties. Mindfulness techniques like deep breathing and meditation can help them stay calm and centered no matter what the school day brings. Teaching children to listen to their friends, teachers, and peers can keep them from feeling out of control or powerless.

Remember that children learn from the adults in their lives, so be an example of someone who stays centered and grounded in the present. If your children see you freaking out and losing control, or stressing over a past regret or a future event, you can guess how they will react in similar situations. Watch your own actions, thoughts, and behaviors, and teach by example the joys of staying mindful.

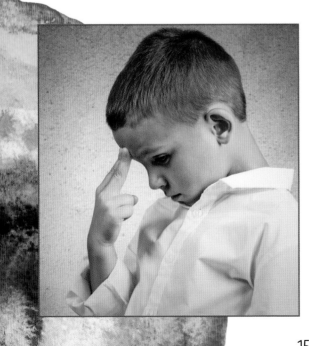

## FRIENDS AND NEIGHBORS

With all the distractions keeping you indoors even on evenings and weekends, it becomes harder to connect with friends or to know your neighbors. Texting and messaging has taken the place of one-on-one time or intimate dinner parties and backyard barbecues on a Sunday afternoon.

Finding time to spend away from technology, television, and social networking enables you to know people in your neighborhood, reconnect with old friends, and cultivate new friendships. Your home is a warm and inviting place where you can bring people in and make them feel acknowledged, heard, and appreciated. Whether you just sit down for a glass of wine with a good friend or cook a lavish dinner for a few couples from down the street, living in the moment opens up new experiences that make you feel less alone and isolated. Bonds are strengthened and even renewed when you step away from addictive texting and other technolgy.

## HAPPIER HOLIDAYS

During the hectic holiday seasons, your home may seem like Grand Central Station, with relatives and friends popping in and out, family staying over and bumping you out of your comfort zone, and constant noise, demands, and distractions that make inner peace impossible.

Much of the chaos you experience over the holidays comes from expectations and frustrations that arise from being around other people. You begin worrying weeks in advance about who will sleep where, what meals you need to prepare, and what gifts you need to buy. Once the holiday is underway, you stress over every aspect of being a good host or guest and rarely enjoy anything. When the holiday is over, you can barely remember what happened because it was such a blur.

Few people get through a major holiday without wanting to cry, scream, break something, or disappear to a tropical island. Mindfulness can not only help you get through the holidays but actually enjoy them and feel more engaged in the good things about spending time with family and friends. It opens you to the idea of doing less and slowing down so you can enjoy the silly stories during dinnertime or be fully engaged in the excitement of children as they open gifts, make cookies, or bask in the warmth of the fire in the fireplace. Fully experience the traditions that

will one day make for the best of memories.

How do you bring mindfulness into one of the most chaotic times of the year? You can start by prioritizing any chores or activities that need to be done before the holidays. Do what you can each day and focus on the task in front of you. If you rush, you miss the joy in the process and risk making mistakes that add to your frustration.

If you are the host or hostess, don't be afraid to excuse yourself for a short meditation in your bathroom or bedroom. If that is impossible, find a quiet corner and do some deep breaths before turning back to your guests. Many times, the person hosting the party enjoys it the least because he or she is so concerned about what can go wrong. Surrender to the moment and have fun, knowing that if something doesn't quite go as planned, you can deal with it from a place of balance and calm.

Mindfulness doesn't have to be about doing anything, though. If you are throwing a party or having your big extended family over for dinner, all it takes is remembering to stop all of the fuss of doing and spend some quality time just being with loved ones. Have fun! Listen to whoever is talking to you, even if it's the aunt you never liked or your awful judgmental neighbor. You may come to find that even the most difficult people have a story to tell and are worthy of your compassion.

If conflicts arise, as they often do, bring out your inner diplomat to explore peaceful resolutions. Holidays are supposed to be about togetherness, food, laughter, and merriment. Get into the music and dance in the kitchen as you stir the sauce. Sit at the kids' table and chat with the young ones about dinosaurs and mermaids. Bring the shy cousin a plate of cookies and ask him about his favorite hobby. Go outside now and then and look at the sunset or the starry night sky. Open yourself to the experience and

be in the moment; when it's time to go back to work or school, everyone will have great memories to share and reminisce about, including you. Time goes by too fast to not give yourself the precious gift of living in the now.

## TROUBLING TIMES

Home isn't always a warm and inviting place. Family conflicts occur, especially when children are involved, or other stressors such as a potential job loss, financial difficulties, death of a pet, aging parents who need care, car problems, and unexpected bills.

Siblings fight. Spouses argue. Teenagers battle with parents. Relatives die.

This is when mindfulness practice is put into action. Whether you do it alone or gather your family together for a deep breathing session, mindful awareness can be a strong and solid foundation from which the problems and challenges of life are approached with greater clarity. That unshakable foundation, found within you and each of your loved ones, provides you with a sacred center to operate from with compassion, empathy, kindness, and diplomacy, rather than the

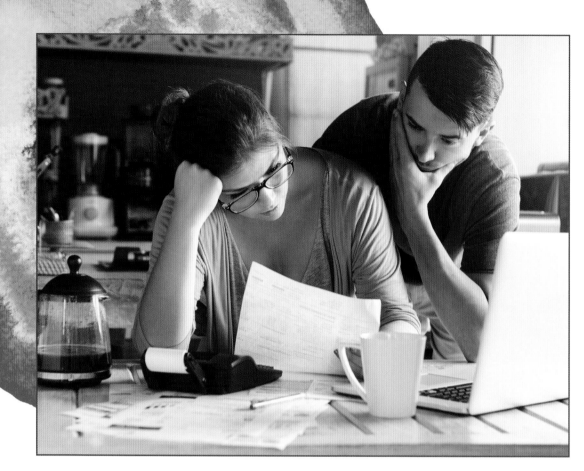

usual knee-jerk anger, fear, and panic-based reactions of the monkey mind.

Tragic events or major accidents will disrupt even the most together, peaceful person, knocking you off your base of equilibrium. Mindfulness can help bring you back to a place of strength and courage, wisdom and insight, and resourcefulness and resilience to navigate the new normal about to unfold around you.

Children are especially fragile during times of conflict. Take your children on a listening walk, a mindful walking meditation that involves you asking them what they see, what they hear, or smell or feel. This focused attention brings them back into the present and clears the worries and fears from their minds, and it gives you a chance to reconnect and show that you are there if and when they need you.

## THE GREATER GOOD

Having a place to call home is about building toward a greater good for all who live under one roof.

Your mindfulness practice contributes to that greater good and can model the behaviors you wish to see in others. If you are calm, cool, and collected, it encourages others to be the same. Home is the good, the bad, and the ugly, but staying present to it all over the chatter and disruptions, both outer and inner, makes for a life worth living and sharing with those you love. Slowing down and paying attention begins in the place you call home, and it spreads to wherever you go once you walk out the door.

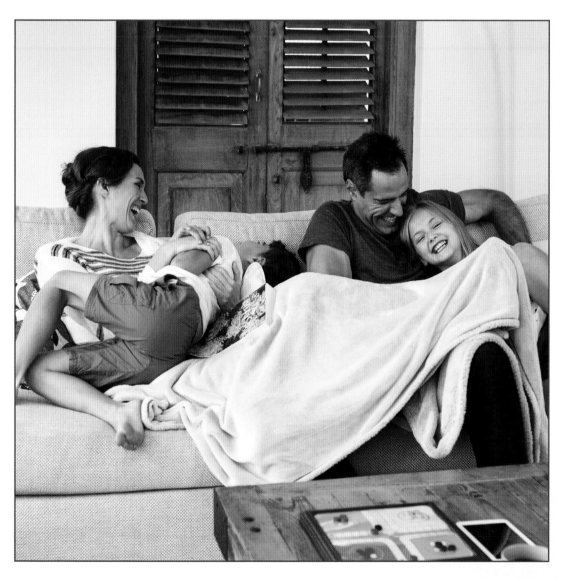

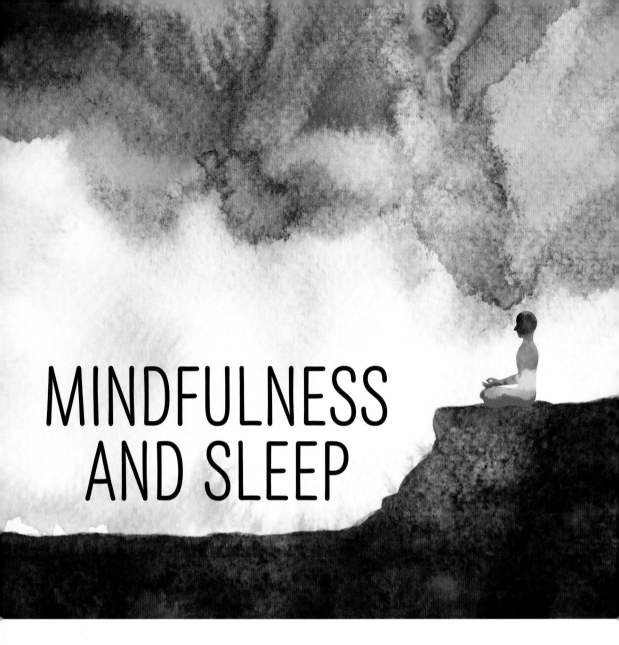

# MINDFULNESS AND SLEEP

Sleep problems affect millions of people of all ages, and they can lead to major health issues if not properly addressed.

You may be able to fall asleep but not stay asleep through the night. Perhaps it takes you hours to relax your body and clear your mind to fall asleep only to find your alarm blaring a few hours later. Lack of sleep doesn't just affect your ability to function the next day: it harms other areas of health and has been linked to a host of diseases and illnesses like obesity and depression.

Bedtime is supposed to be a time to cast aside the concerns of the day, but if your mind is filled with worry and anxiety about finances, children, spouses, jobs, or a host of other things, it can become a nightmare. You feel anxious about not being able to sleep, which makes sleep more elusive. Once you add the growing addiction to digital devices, relaxation and rest become even more elusive. The mind never stops focusing on "doing," and you become tempted to manage sleeplessness with a pill or medication.

## MINDFUL SCIENCE

Whether you have full-blown insomnia or just an occasional sleepless night, mindfulness can help, and there is ample science to back up this claim. One study, featured in *The Journal of the American Medical Association* in February 2015, examined the effects of mindfulness on middle-aged and older adults with sleeping difficulties. The small clinical trial took 49 participants (with an average age of 65) and separated them into two groups. The first group went through a mindfulness program called MAP,

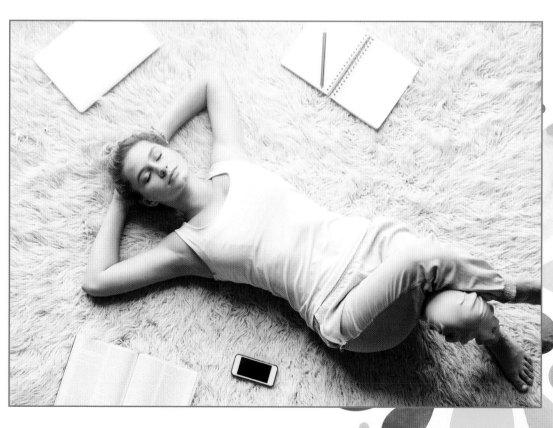

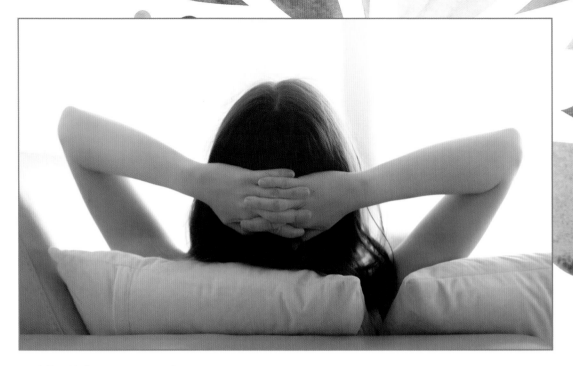

or Mindful Awareness Program, using meditation and exercises to help them focus on their present-moment thoughts, emotions, and experiences. The second group completed a SHE, or Sleep Hygiene Education, a more intellectual approach focused on improving sleep habits.

The two groups each met once a week for a two-hour period six times. By the end of the six sessions, the mindfulness group reported less fatigue and insomnia than the other group; the mindfulness group's depression and anxiety levels also decreased. The end result was that mindfulness had a strong role in positively addressing sleep problems in older adults.

Herbert Benson, Director Emeritus of the Harvard-affiliated Benson-Henry Institute for Mind Body Medicine, coined the phrase "relaxation response," a physiological shift that is the exact opposite of the stress response. The relaxation response reduces not only stress and worry but pain, high blood pressure, and other blocks to a good night's sleep. Benson recommends daily meditation that focuses on the breath and keeps the mind present, allowing worries of the past and future to drift by without reaction or response. You can even use a mantra or sound, a short prayer or positive quote, or any other aid to help the mind from engaging in needless worry.

In a 2015 study conducted by Ute Hülsheger, an associate professor of work and organizational psychology at the Maastricht University in the Netherlands, participants read materials about mindfulness and then took part in exercises, including breathing, body scans, and loving-kindness meditation. The two-week program asked participants to meditate using different combinations of the exercises for just 10 minutes a day, before and after work. There were also questionnaires to fill out in the morning, after work, and at bedtime to gauge sleep quality and the ability to detach from work-related worries.

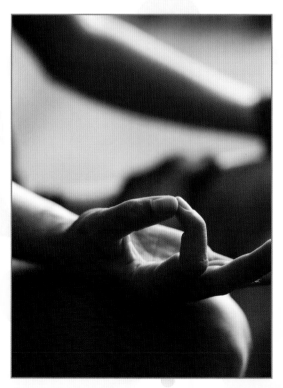

Results showed marked improvement in sleep quality and sleep duration, although more intensive training was required to learn the art of detaching from work thoughts and concerns. However, Hülsheger stated that practicing mindfulness exercises for a short duration would not keep the sleep issues from returning, and that regular ongoing mindfulness practice provided the most sustainable positive effects.

Mindfulness must become a lifestyle if sleep disturbances are to be permanently eradicated. But the truth is, you don't have to exhaust yourself in an intensive practice that leaves you more exhausted than when you began. It just has to be consistent.

Work stress isn't the only enemy of healthy sleep. Family and home life, school pressure, financial concerns, and physical health issues all serve to prevent you from experiencing the kind of rejuvenating sleep you need. Even a quick worry detox before bed in the form of deep breathing and focused meditation helps soothe the chaotic, overactive mind to improve sleep.

Besides having a mindfulness practice during the day, creating a program before bedtime that suits you is critical to allowing the mind to

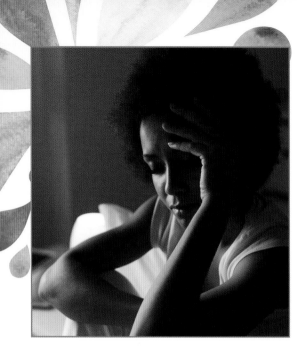

turn down the "inner noise volume" and prepare for rest. You will sleep better and experience better focus and memory, reduced stress, less mental rumination, more clarity, improved energy levels, and positive benefits to your relationships with others. Restorative sleep can do wonders for your mood, and it can lessen anger, frustration, and hostility at work and at home.

Before you get into bed, complete a sitting meditation. It doesn't have to be longer than 10 minutes. Sit in a comfortable place and keep the mind focused on breathing or a mantra, allowing thoughts to drift in and out without attachment or concern. Notice each body part, and pay attention to areas where you might need to release tension. Breathe in and out, and bring your mind back to the breath should it wander. When you feel relaxed, open your eyes and get into bed.

Once you are in bed, if you continue to feel agitation and tension, you can either get up and complete another short meditation or close your eyes and focus on a mantra or image until sleep comes. When uncomfortable thoughts appear, you can acknowledge them with love and compassion. You can say, "I acknowledge these fears of not having enough money to pay the bills, thank you." Allow the thought to move along as if on a conveyor belt.

## FROM DOING TO BEING

Mindfulness before bedtime escorts the mind from doing to being. You may want to employ a visual guided meditation geared toward transitioning the mind of goal-based, results-oriented thoughts and into a state of pure awareness.

Doing doesn't just refer to physical actions. Ruminating over something you did wrong, or need to do in the future, is also an act of "doing" because you are engaged in the action of obsessing over something you have no control of in the present moment.

There is plenty of time during the day to focus on goals and directives. Make sure you don't bring that doingness into the bedroom when it's time to put an end to the day and transition into a state conducive to sleeping well.

You may have trouble staying in the present moment because it doesn't feel productive; however, mindfulness benefits more than just your boss's to-do list or your wallet. It benefits your health, well-being, and capacity for happiness and fulfillment in a world that too often measures success on a monetary scale or by the number of items you crossed off your achievement list.

Living in the present is the only time you truly experience life. Through mindfulness, you end up feeling more fulfilled, more accomplished, and more engaged with life. The focus turns away from rushing to do as many things as you can cram into a few hours to being alive and open to the sensations and experiences as they happen.

## STEPS TO SLEEP

Make mindfulness practice a nighttime routine by having your own method of putting the day to rest. You can always switch up the techniques you employ over time, but the routine should be carved in stone on your calendar. A half hour before bedtime is all you need, but make it consistent and let family members know they are

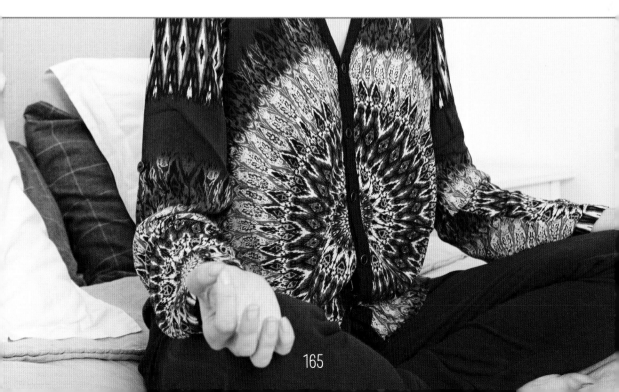

not to interrupt you unless it's an emergency. If family members see you sleeping better, it will inspire them to create their own bedtime practice, too.

Impose a no-work rule and stick to it. This may mean no work after 6 p.m., or you can stop all at-home work before dinner. You may be tempted to continue working, but the mind, like the body, needs time to decompress and switch off.

Make sure your room and sleeping environment are free of clutter. It may sound painfully obvious, but if you are trying to sleep on a too-

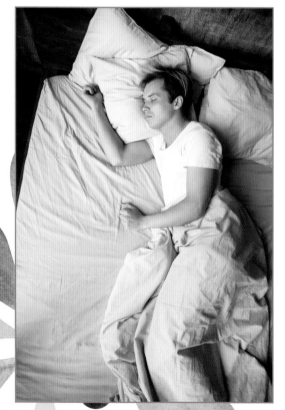

soft or too-hard mattress, or in a position that doesn't support your head, neck, and spine, quality sleep will elude you. Your bedroom should be a retreat and a place you look forward to at the end of a long day and not the cause of more stress.

Dress for bed in comfortable and unrestricting clothing. Keep your bedroom cool, as cooler temperatures are more conducive to sleep. If you use a fan, try to find a low-noise model.

Turn off all electronics before you get into bed, and keep room lighting as low as possible. If you must keep a cell phone on, move it to where you won't be tempted to keep looking at it, and adjust the screen light to the lowest setting.

If you wish, have a cup of soothing, decaffeinated tea before you begin your meditation. You can look for specific herbal teas beneficial to relaxation and sleep, such as chamomile, valerian, passionflower, lemon balm or decaffeinated green teas. There are also many lines of sleepytime or nighttime teas, but make sure to check that they don't interfere with medications or existing issues like high blood pressure or diabetes.

You can play soft, relaxing music, so long as it does not distract you from your meditation. You may find music helps calm the monkey chatter in your mind much easier than total silence. The music shouldn't have loud sounds, drums, or horns.

For especially challenging days, you may want to start with a warm bubble bath. Light some candles and put on soothing music. Feel the warmth of the water melt away the problems of the day. Let it all rinse off the body and mind like water down the drain.

Stretching is a great way to get the body loose and relaxed. Even a few yoga poses geared toward removing tension and resistance can help assist in preparing for sleep, so long as you are not working up a sweat or exerting too much energy. Going to bed with stiff muscles or body aches is a surefire way to disrupt sleep. A stretching routine keeps you from depending on pills and drugs that only serve to add to restless and interrupted sleep with side effects like dry mouth and morning grogginess.

Focus on your breath. This is a superb mindfulness activity and a part of any mindfulness practice you choose. It increases oxygen and blood flow to the brain and the vital organs. Shallow chest breathing brings about chest tension and tightness in the abdominal area.

Breathe deeply into the belly area, hold the breath, and then release slowly.

## EXTRA TRICKS FOR RESTFUL SLEEP

Progressive muscle relaxation engages both body and mind to relax each muscle group and eliminate tension. The process is simple but requires focus.

Start with each specific body part and tighten the muscles to a count of five and release. Move on to the next body part, tightening and releasing until your whole body feels free from tension and resistance.

Start with your toes. Focus your mind as you wiggle them; tighten them by curling them as hard as you can. Hold them for five seconds, and then release and wiggle them again. Flex the foot back tightly for five seconds and then release it.

Eventually you can move to the ankles, shins, thighs, groin, buttocks, abdomen, fingers, hands, arms, shoulders, chest, neck, and face. You will feel heavy as you let each muscle group relax. That means you are doing the progression correctly.

You may notice particular parts of the body that seem more resistant

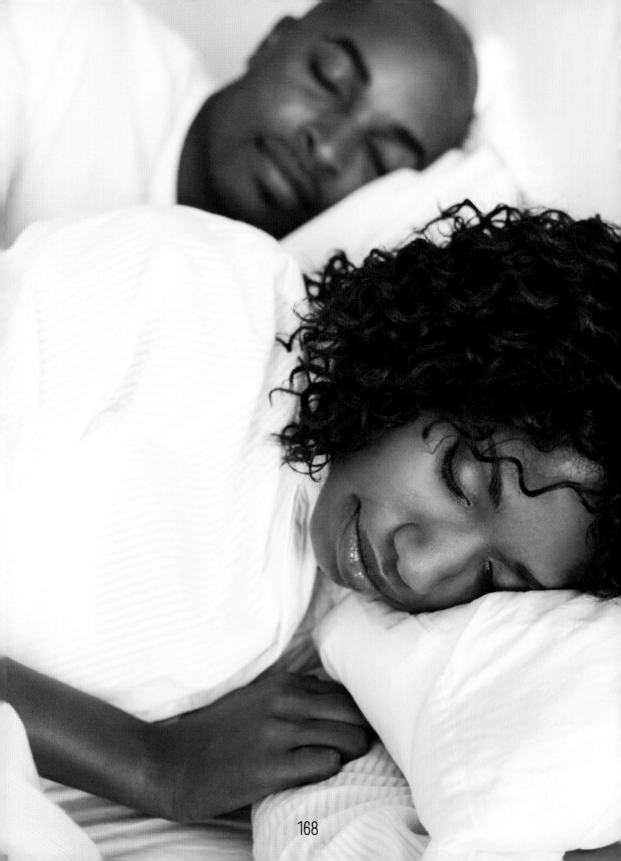

and require extra attention. Don't be afraid to go back and complete another squeeze-and-release, keeping the mind fully present to the sensations of the muscles flexing and relaxing. Once the body sinks into the bed, heavy and free, you can follow this up with deep breathing, keeping your mind focused as you inhale and exhale until you fall asleep.

Aromatherapy is another sleep aid that can be used in conjunction with your breathing exercise or meditation. Certain smells relax and soothe when inhaled directly; they can be used in diffusers, added to warm evening baths, or spritzed on pillowcases and bed linens. You can use a few drops of oil on a cotton ball and place it near your pillow. Look for essential oils known for promoting sleep and calm, and don't be afraid to try a few to see what you like best.

Lavender essential oil is the most popular, because of its properties for calming the mind while also bringing a sense of clarity. You can spritz lavender directly onto your pillowcase or place a lavender cache beneath your pillow. Diluted oils can be dabbed on the wrists or neck as well. Frankincense is another

calming oil that rids the body and mind of anxiety and stress. If you feel agitated and ungrounded, look for marjoram, vetiver, cedarwood, or neroli oils.

Though the use of aromatherapy is not a cure for sleeplessness, it is a tool that assists the body and mind to relax and fall asleep faster. Be careful not to choose stimulating scents like cypress, peppermint, lemon, or grapefruit that will counteract your attempts and make you feel too energetic for sleep. You can learn about aromatherapy online or visit a local qualified aromatherapy practitioner to find the scent that is perfect for your needs.

Nighttime is supposed to be a time of peace, calm, and rest. Mindfulness practices such as meditation serve to quiet the daily chatter of memories, negative self-talk, judgments, blame, anger, and frustration so that you wake up restored, refreshed, and ready to face the new day.

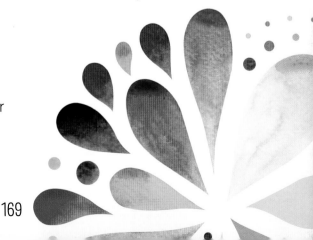

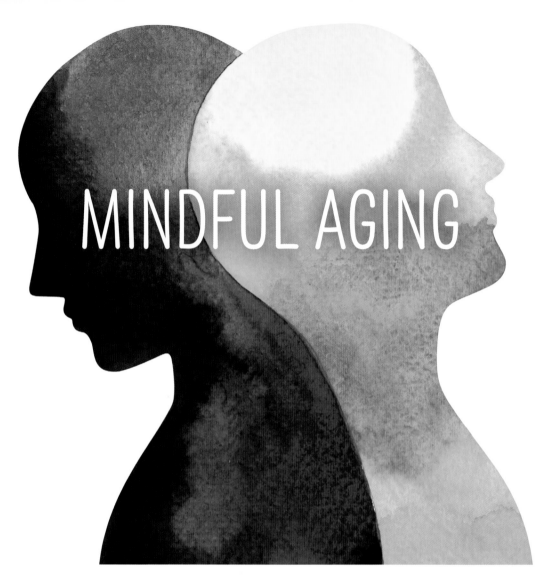

# MINDFUL AGING

Few people like to think about aging. The truth is, you start growing older from the moment you are born, and you can either consider it a blessing or a curse.

Not everyone has the luxury of living a long, fulfilling life. Some people die young; others live to over 100 years old. Due to illnesses that steal vitality and mental clarity, some people die in spirit long before their bodies perish, while others are productive into their 90s.

Time goes by fast. In the blink of an eye, you go from a happy-go-lucky child to a busy adult with a job, spouse, house, and children of your own. It happens so quickly that you don't realize it until something like an illness or tragedy shakes you out of your daily complacency and reminds you of the ticking clock of mortality. Then you suddenly awaken to the lost years you spent worrying and stressing, so focused on the past and future, you forgot about the gifts of the present.

## GIFTS OF AGING

There is no way you will recognize the gifts of aging if you are trapped in fear and resentment of the process. By changing your perspective, you can begin to feel grateful for every day you awake. Gratitude is a mindfulness exercise itself, because when you are thankful, you are automatically aware of the positive things you have. Keeping a gratitude journal and writing down five things you are grateful for each day directs you to the blessings that illuminate your life.

It is impossible to be in a thankful state when you are angry or afraid. Journaling connects you to your inner thoughts and feelings; you can explore the fears you have over mortality, diminishing health, and losing loved ones. You cannot escape from the cycle of life, aging, and death, but becoming mindful of your deepest fears allows you to face them and lessen their negative and destructive power.

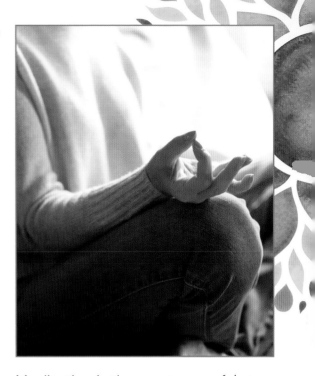

Meditation is the most powerful mindfulness exercise to bring clarity to the mind so that the challenges of aging can be faced with compassion and courage. Meditation trains you to focus on the everyday things you rush past in your quest to get more done or finish your to-do list. These daily activities may not seem important at the time, but in the years to come, you will look back and wish you had slowed down and lived them more presently and fully, especially those moments involving your loved ones.

No one wishes to be old; nevertheless, older people consistently poll the highest in happiness levels. Age brings wisdom, including the ability to recognize that each moment, no matter how boring or trivial, is a moment to be cherished, because it will never come back again. Moments turn into days, weeks, months, and years; when you live your life on autopilot trapped in a loop of past and future worries, you wake up one day filled with painful regret for "what might have been."

## THE AGING BRAIN

Mindfulness protects the brain from losing focus, flexibility, and cognitive capacity. Memory loss and degrading cognitive performance can be diminished by practicing meditation, for meditation helps to maintain mental acuity and neuroplasticity, which is the ability of the adult brain to keep learning and changing as it ages. The idea is to keep your "neural reserve" in great working order. This reserve refers to your brain's mental capacity, efficiency, and flexibility.

A 2017 study in the *Journal of Cognitive Enhancement* titled "Meditation and Cognitive Ageing: The Role of Mindfulness Meditation in Building Cognitive Reserve" examined the ways meditation practices engaged cognitive skills associated with focus and sustained attention. Mindfulness meditation slowed down cognitive decline and actually increased neural processes and cognitive reserve capacity.

Another study published in *Frontiers in Psychology* in September 2014 examined a number of research studies covering the various forms of meditation and their effects on brain function and capacity. The study team found that different types of mindfulness meditation could lead to improvement in different neural structures and brain activity. The team found meditation reduces stress, affects the way the brain perceives and processes the world, and strengthens focus and concentration.

Using your brain keeps it working better as you age. There are a plethora of brain exercises, games, and puzzles, but mindfulness activates brain networks that can help with creativity, sharpen attention to detail, and enhance memory. Because older brains are often less flexible, thoughts become more rigid, fixed, and resistant to new ideas and opinions. Meditation emphasizes a deeper awareness of thoughts, feelings, and sensation free from judgment and criticism. The result is a more open, flexible mind that sees new ideas and perspectives like that of a much younger person.

Mindfulness decreases attachment

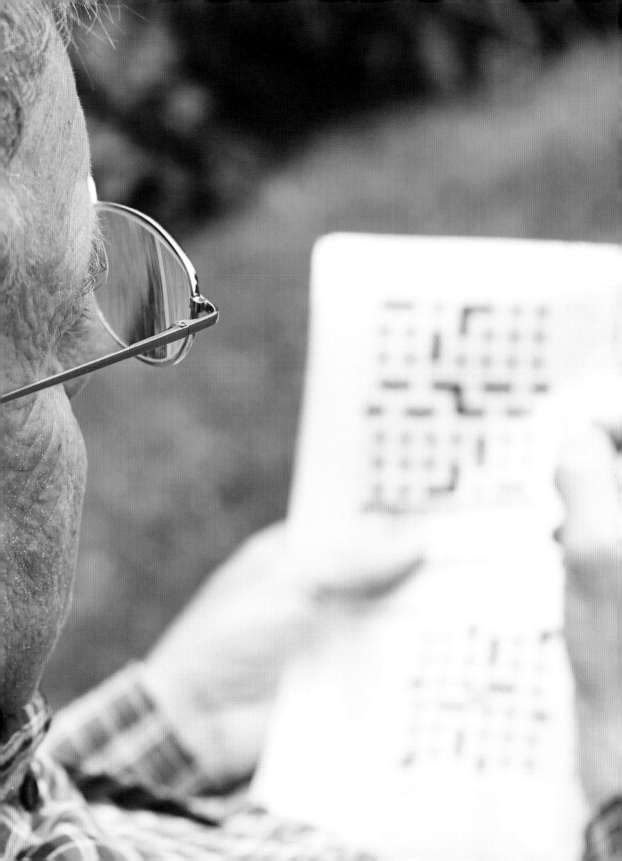

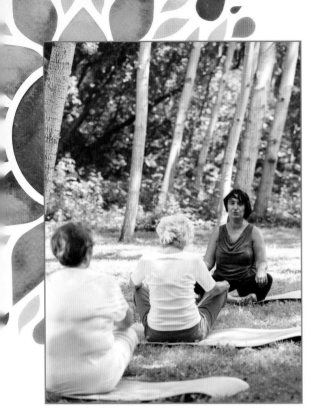

Shook and her colleagues at West Virginia University explored the idea of a "well-being paradox" that suggests people become more mindful naturally with age and thus report feeling better about life than their more stressed and younger counterparts.

Shook's study involved 123 adults between ages 25 and 35, and 117 older adults between ages 60 and 91. They all lived in the same area, and a majority of the adults were female. The participants were asked questions about their mood, mindfulness, and perspective of the future, as well as their current positive and negative emotions. They also were asked how much they stayed mindful to the awareness of the moment instead of living in the past or anticipating the future.

to specific ways of being, thinking, and doing. Aging people often hang tightly on to traditions and beliefs that no longer serve them, for they lack the actual mental acuity and capacity to see life from a different angle. Mindfulness increases that acuity and capacity, adding to the richness of life even in the later years.

## THE WELL-BEING PARADOX

Not every aging person becomes rigid and regretful. Look at the many older artists, writers, actors, musicians, business owners, and athletes that defy the stereotypes of old age. A study by Natalie J.

The study's results showed the older adults were more aware of the fact that they had fewer remaining years to live and felt more positive emotions because of their focus on the here and now. Compared to the younger adults, the older group lived with greater mindfulness, which translated to greater well-being. Shook wrote in her study that the "cultivation of mindfulness may be an adaptive means of maintaining emotional well-being when faced with life's challenges." This positive spin on life, often prompted by an awareness of mortality, can lead to improved physical health.

The older group's shift of the perspective of time is in direct opposition to the "all the time in the world" perspective of the younger group and may be the key to mindfulness and more happiness in the later years. By embracing old age, rather than denying and shunning it, you can experience a full life.

## THE TELOMERE CONNECTION

Can mindfulness actually slow the aging process on a genetic level? The answer is yes, according to the work of Elizabeth H. Blackburn of the University of California, San Francisco. Blackburn and her colleagues won a Nobel Prize in 2009 for the discovery of telomerase, a protective enzyme found in your cells that replenishes and lengthens telomeres.

Telomeres are the protective tips or caps at the end of chromosomes. They help cells divide in a healthy manner; as cells divide, telomeres become shorter in length. Eventually, the cell dies. Research shows that telomerase can replenish telomeres and even re-lengthen them; this results in a healthier cell life.

Stress is associated with shorter telomere length, as are diseases associated with aging like cancer, diabetes, heart disease, and osteoporosis. Chronic stress shortens telomeres, too, as well as pessimism, worry, and depression. These mental states cause your cells and your body to age more rapidly. This may explain why two people the same age can look so different physically. One may have longer telomeres and a much more positive attitude and mental state, which leads to more longer telomeres and thus a healthier mind and body.

Can mindfulness and other practices lengthen and strengthen telomeres? Again, the answer is yes. In several

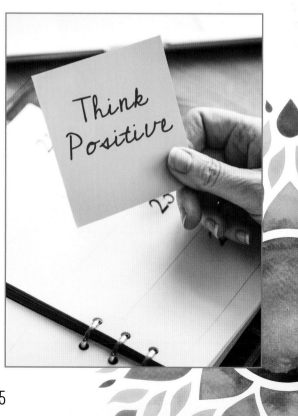

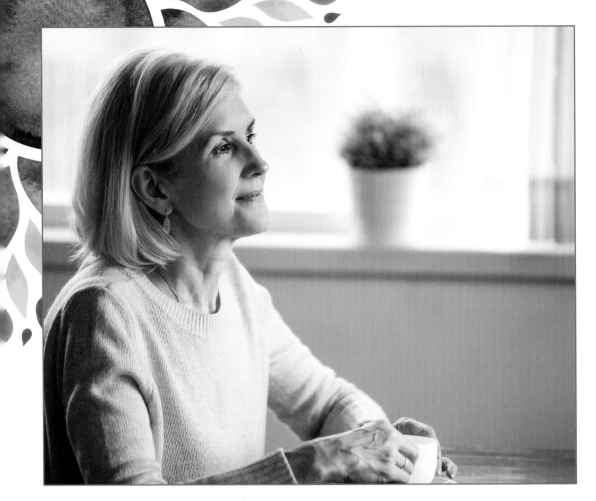

studies, including one by Clifford Saron of the Center for Mind and Brain at the University of California, Davis, meditation was found to promote positive psychological changes. Another study by Elissa Epel and her colleagues in the *Annals of the New York Academy of Sciences* in 2009 showed that even a wandering mind leads to shorter telomeres.

## POSITIVE AGING

The key to all of this is mindfulness. Mindfulness also improves health on the chromosomal level. Mindfulness not only makes the brain more flexible and youthful, but it encourages the adaptive regulation of emotion and reactivity.

Much of your fear and concerns about aging may come from media and social media, where youth and young bodies are celebrated, worshipped, and adored. This youth-centric focus is not only destructive, but it is ridiculous, for even the youngest among us will age. If you feel you are having difficulty facing aging because of the media, news, advertising, social media, or any other external factor, find ways to remove yourself from the flow of negativity. Unplug for short or even long periods of time.

There are plenty of websites, social networking groups, books, movies, television shows, and other media that celebrate age. Seek them out. You might even look at how other cultures treat their elderly. You'd be surprised to see many countries and traditions revere their senior citizens and look to them for guidance and direction.

Being mindful means having your own perceptions and perspectives of what it means to age, regardless of the thoughts and complaints of those around you. Remove yourself from friends and colleagues that continuously complain about their aches and pains and downsides of each passing year. Celebrate every birthday with joy and gratitude for having another circle around the sun. Look for positive influences in the seniors around you that you can model.

Above all, be mindful that the more time you spend hating the fact you are getting older, the more time you lose over something you cannot stop. But you can control your response to it: you can turn it from a negative and disabling response to a positive and enthusiastic one.

With each passing year, science and research teach us more about the aging process and how your diet, exercise plan, and emotional states affect the way you age. You have the choice to make decisions that benefit your health and increase your chances of entering your golden years feeling golden. Or you can go in kicking, screaming, and resisting the natural cycle of life.

Age doesn't have to mean pain, suffering, or decline. Engaging the mind and body in mindfulness practices brings back a youthful energy and quality to life; it also teaches you to accept the reality of aging. It even helps you embrace the good things about growing old, such as greater wisdom, compassion, understanding, and self-awareness. Youth is wonderful, but age can be just as grand a time if you stay present to what it has to offer, including the miracle of being able to get up and live another day full of possibility and promise.

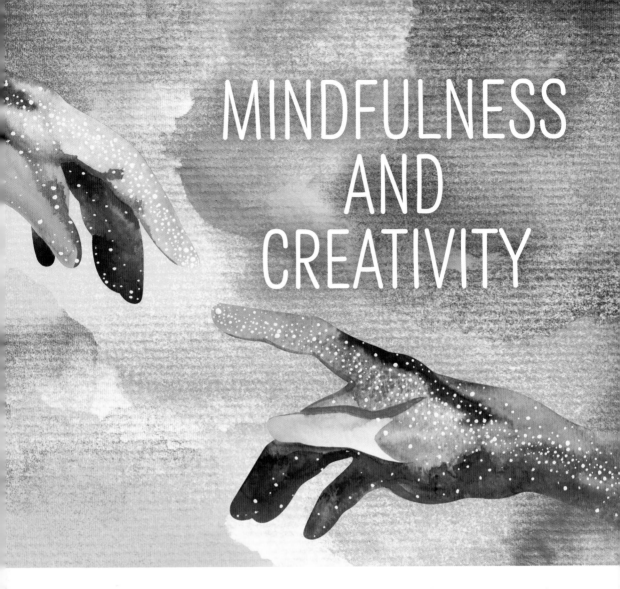

# MINDFULNESS AND CREATIVITY

Whether you engage in creative activity for fun or make a living out of it, the creative process involves finding ways to express oneself without becoming immobilized by self-judgment, criticism, or fear. For the lucky few, being creative comes naturally; for most, it isn't something that feels natural at all, and it often demands breaking through deep-rooted self-consciousness, subconscious blocks, and inner fears about the act of expressing oneself through art, music, writing, or any other creative endeavor.

Even if you aren't planning to paint a portrait or write a novel, increasing creativity can benefit all areas of your life, including your job and family responsibilities. When you must make a decision, find a

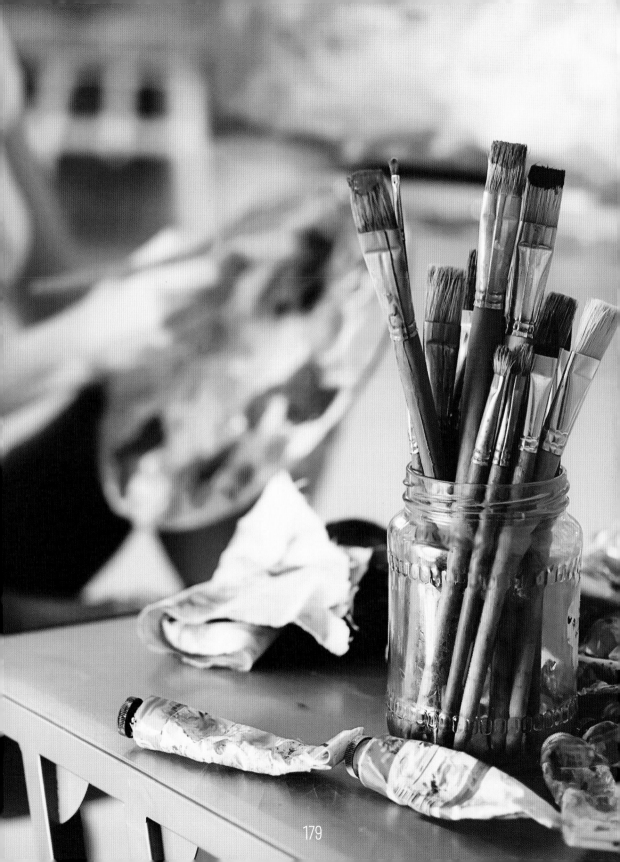

solution to a problem, or brainstorm an outside-the-box way to do something different, creativity is involved. Mindfulness opens the door to innovative ideas and solutions that you may never have thought of before; it also provides new perspectives on tricky problems.

The biggest block to creativity is fear. Fear of being judged. Fear of failing. Fear of looking foolish or wasting time that could be used for more "rational" acts like laundry and working. Fear of exposure and vulnerability. By becoming aware of negative or judgmental thoughts, you provide room for creativity to grow. And when both sides of the brain are actively engaged—the analytical and rational left brain and the sensory and impressionable right brain—you can make art.

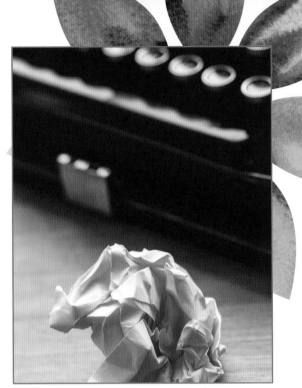

## MEDITATING AND THE CREATIVE PROCESS

The word "creativity" means to bring about something that was not there before. Sometimes a creative concept comes in a flash of brilliance, but for most people, it is a process. You know this process well if you've ever created so much as a high school essay or an art project.

It starts with preparation. In his 1926 book *The Art of Thought*,

Graham Wallas, the cofounder of the London School of Economics, formulated a four-step plan to train the mind in the art of creativity. Those four steps are:

**Preparation**
**Incubation**
**Illumination**
**Verification**

**Preparation** quiets the part of the brain that engages in cognitive thinking.

**Incubation** involves occupying yourself with mundane activities while the mind organizes and examines. Think of it as going "offline" so you can step back and enter a calm state of mind.

**Illumination** brings about a powerful insight or "aha" moment of recognition. Many people ascribe "aha" moments to the time their reality and their intuition come into alignment.

**Verification** is a final reality check. In this final step, you allow cognitive thinking to shape your idea into something that is born.

Being mindful to the flow of ideas is a must to begin, and sustain, the entire creative process. Meditation is the tool that keeps the channels open; ideally, the flow continues when you are faced with repeated fears and doubts. Undoubtedly, some people may be more naturally creative than others and have to work at those steps with less effort.

## THE END

Here are three words to know: excuses, noise, and distractions.

These three words are enemies of creativity. Mindful creativity is more than merely arriving at new ideas. It is about an ongoing battle against the old habits that inhibit your creativity, those destructive habits that you fall back on subconsciously.

Excuses are based upon fear of outcomes. You don't want to write because you feel tired and need a nap. The outcome of writing and the

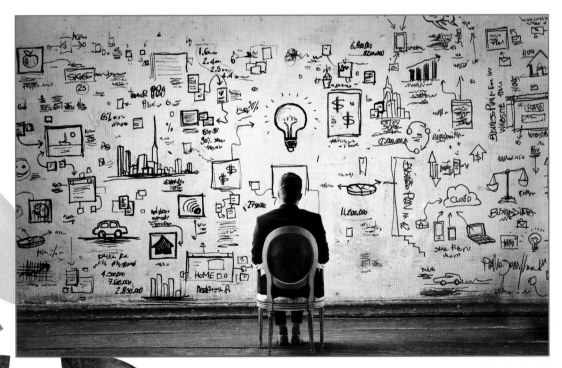

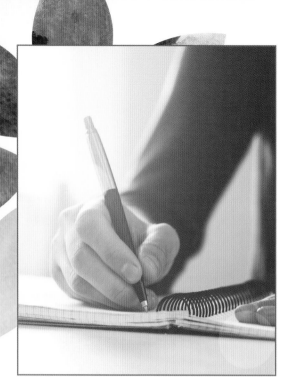

the task is a creative one. Without discipline, you will be scattered with your time and thoughts. Meditation disciplines the mind to let go of attachments to particular thoughts and the judgments that accompany them—the perfect situation for innovative thinking to take root.

## ENGAGING THE SENSES

You see, hear, feel, touch, and smell. But how often during the course of an average day do you really notice what your five senses are experiencing? Mindfulness puts you back in control, allowing you to really see, hear, feel, touch, and smell what is in front of you and enjoy the experience. Being fully present cultivates mindfulness because you are so engaged in the moment at hand, and how your body is responding to it, that you have no time to think of anything else.

challenges it brings, not to mention the vulnerability of exposing your storytelling abilities on paper, result in you finding something else that you should do instead, even something rational like catching up on sleep.

Any writer or artist will tell you that each day brings a new set of issues to overcome. Building a mindfulness practice around a creative pursuit will include building new habits to replace the old and eliminate the END.

Having discipline may seem like it has no place in the free-for-all world of creativity, but discipline provides the perfect foundation to keep you focused and on task, even when

All five senses are firing on all cylinders, clearing the mind of unnecessary clutter; when this happens, creativity is born and nurtured. The mind becomes fully present and aware of its surroundings. It's hard to be worried about bills that need to be paid, or a work project with a looming deadline, when you are in a setting that awakens your senses and makes you feel alive. Yet even if you cannot leave your desk and run outside to take a "nature break," you can certainly sit and meditate. You can visualize a warm summer day and bring your mind back from the edge of chaos to the sacred center within where calmness prevails.

## DEFAULT MODE

Neuroscientists often consider a default mode of the brain that is conducive to creativity. It may sound counterintuitive, but this default mode is free of any external focus or interference and is referred to as a state of wakeful rest. You may argue and say focus is needed for creativity, and you would be right.

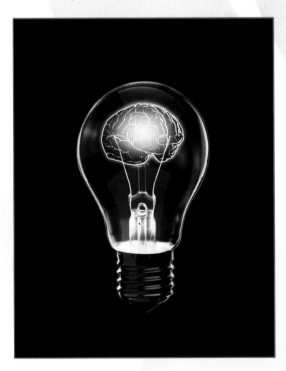

But the brain must first free itself from outer-directed thoughts in order to find that inner focus. You function in this default mode when you are not worrying about the past or future.

Were it not for this default mode, you would never notice how scrumptious your mom's homemade chocolate chip cookies are—how they melt in your mouth and remind you of your childhood. No matter the size and scope of your creative endeavor, the default mode is where you find a calm place and welcome the gifts of introspection.

Have you ever found yourself staring at something for an hour and feeling as though you left your body? You became so focused on that one thing, say a rock or a piece of note paper, that you got lost and "forgot yourself." This is much different from rumination, where your mind enters a destructive and time-wasting loop, repeating the same thoughts over and over again until you feel obsessed and desperate for relief.

Daydreams are a form of mindfulness meditation involving visualizations of what you wish would happen. Even though you are imagining a future event or replaying a past one, the act of daydreaming removes you from the restrictions of body and brain and allows your

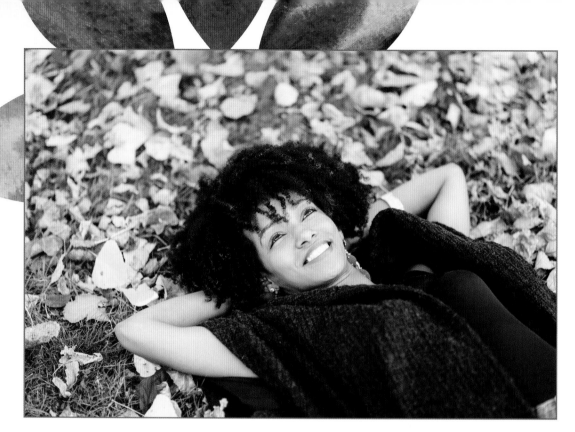

mind to create a new reality where you are dreaming about what is really happening. Daydreaming is incredibly conducive to creative thinking: it allows the mind to go beyond limitations and restrictions of "reality," like a nighttime dream.

## CREATIVITY AT WORK

You don't have to be a novelist or artist to call yourself creative. Any job imaginable has room for the creative process and can benefit from cultivating creative thinking. You may work at a mortgage firm, a warehouse, or even a big box store; no matter where you work, you can find ways to incorporate creativity into your job. Being creative at work is a must if you feel stuck in your job or blocked on a solution to a certain problem. Difficult projects become more enjoyable and conquerable with creative thinking. You might even come up with a few ideas that generate larger profits and more productivity.

Tried-and-true often works on the job, but there is always room for new ideas. Feeling stifled and suppressed because "this is how it's always been done" keeps you, your coworkers, and your company from growing and thriving. When the workplace becomes fun, everyone can benefit.

Being at work often requires that you find ways to balance various parts of the brain that could make or break your on-the-job experience. You know being too emotional and reactive at work can get you into trouble, so using mindfulness techniques is a great way to maintain peace and balance. If all emotion is kept out of the process, you end up with a cold, robotic workplace and a stifled environment with little room for fresh ideas.

The oldest part of the brain is the reptilian brain, and it only concerned with your survival. The reptilian brain focuses on whether or not you should fight, or take flight, in a given situation; it has little room or time for creativity. It is fixed on keeping you alive. Without this part of the brain, survival would be threatened, but if you only operate from the reptilian brain, you are not going to be able to see anything outside of a very small box you need to stay in for your own safety and protection. At work, reacting from this brain leads to extreme competitiveness, an inability to compromise, and hostility toward your coworkers.

The different parts of the brain all work together to make us function at our best, with one area kicking in when needed and others taking a backseat until they are called upon to perform their specific duties. With mindfulness meditation or any other

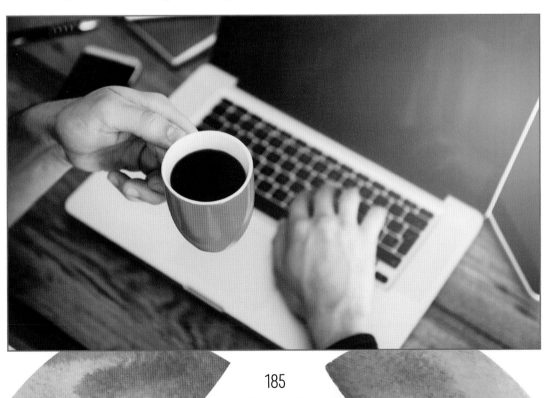

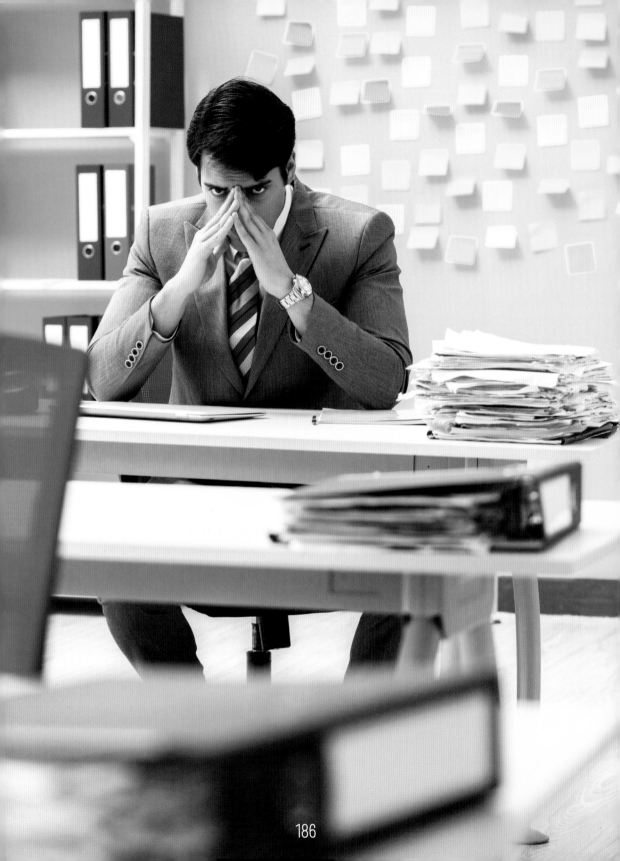

practice, you can achieve a state of quiet and calm alertness that overrides any one particular part of the brain going haywire and causing strife, conflict, and discord.

Meditation erodes cognitive rigidity. Cognitive rigidity is valuable when you need to hunt to feed your family or evade warring tribes, but it isn't as prized in a job where you need to work with other people toward a common goal.

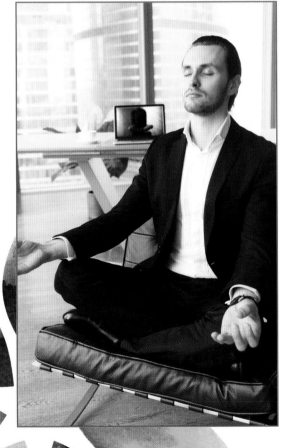

## INNOVATION

Innovation drives many companies to come up with amazing new products, services, and goods. It also works at home when you are trying to figure out ways to entertain three kids and make dinner at the same time. Need drives innovation, but creativity offers the sources of ideas from which innovative products and services spring forth. A problem can never be solved at the same level of thinking that created it in the first place. It requires going "above and beyond" the problem itself to seek new perspectives, visions, and solutions.

Pick a particular problem you've been struggling with. Meditate on it daily, allowing the mind to stay clear of judgment or pressure, and no doubt you will think of the perfect solution in the shower or on the freeway three days later (after it has time to incubate). This is because the mind has obtained the gift of clarity; without clarity, the mind cannot create.

Every wonderful product or service you use was once the creative thought in the mind of someone who recognized how innovative it was. They saw a need and arrived at a new and exciting way to fill that need. Creativity is about more than making a pretty picture. It's about making new things that did not exist before, whether it's a new way to make coffee, a more absorbent diaper, or a window shade that rises and drops with the snap of a finger.

Does mindfulness really boost creativity? Yes, according to a study involving 129 participants in an experiment performed at Erasmus University in the Netherlands. Participants were divided into three groups and told to generate as many business ideas involving drones as possible. One group completed a 10-minute guided meditation before they began. The second group completed a fake meditation during which they were told to think freely and let their minds wander. The third group went to work brainstorming without any meditation.

Even though all three groups came up with the same number of ideas, the guided meditation group came up with a wider range of ideas that

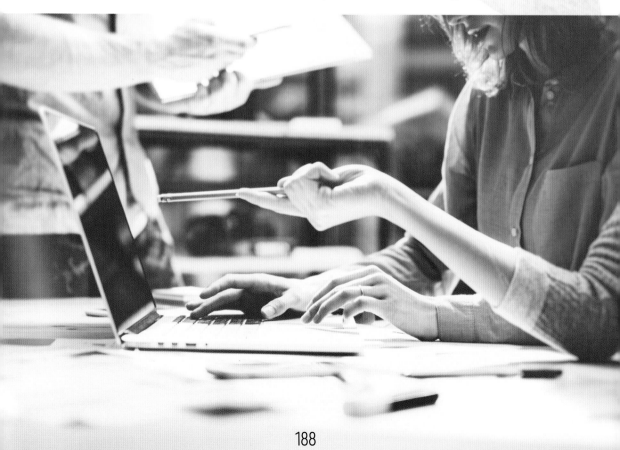

spanned more categories. The guided meditation gave this group more mental clarity, flexibility, and positivity. Meditation also decreased the anxiety and irritation levels of the group compared to the other two groups.

Meditation in the workplace results in calmer, more creative employees who are able to come up with a diverse number of ideas.

## MAKING THINGS

Creativity is a part of the human experience, whether you do it for fun or for work. First, you must move past the formidable gatekeepers that make you want to give up before you can even begin.

In order to let your creative juices flow, it would be ideal to have plenty of alone time, free from distractions; however, that is not always possible. To let the ideas loose, complete a meditation beforehand. If you don't have time to meditate or are not in a place conducive for it, a few deep belly breaths can prepare the mind for creative pursuits.

Perhaps you don't have the best supplies or space for making art. This is just another excuse! Any place can be a perfect place if you want it to be. You may not have room in your house to set up a woodworking shop, but how about a dedicated space in your garage?

Creativity is usually associated with having the luxury of not working, of being "lazy" and unproductive. How many times have you said to yourself, "I don't have time to be creative. I have to __." If you have time to watch television or nose through your cell phone for hours, you have time to be creative.

## INSPIRATION

Even if you are not feeling inspired, you can use mindfulness to find your flow and, subsequently, inspiration.

The word "inspired" means to "breathe into." Being inspired, and acting on it right away, is ideal, but when life is bearing down on you, often the last thing you feel is that sense of connectedness to something greater than yourself that breathes into you a wonderful idea for self-expression.

Anyone can be creative, and anyone can be inspired to create by doing a few simple things. Becoming playful and open to life is critical, unless you want to make angry art. Becoming centered and clear so ideas can pop up in the field of your mind plants the seeds for some of those ideas to grow into full-blown works of art or amazing and useful solutions. Meditating for awareness and focus keeps the mind from monkey chatter and useless ruminating and brings it back to the present. Finding more creativity in your life can inspire you to strengthen the creative muscles.

## CHILDREN AND CREATIVITY

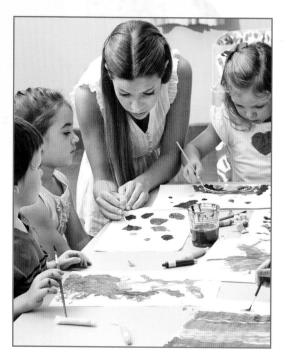

Find time to allow your child to explore his or her creativity. Life isn't simply about school, rules, or chores. Children need to express themselves, and they love to do that by making things. They paint, they play games, they dance, they make up stories, they learn instruments, they sing, and they imagine. These are gifts that many adults sadly lose sight of once "maturity" sets in. Children are often drawn to a particular means of self-expression, and that should be nurtured and cultivated. There are many classes and pastimes in your neighborhood, as well as online activities, that can expose your child to creative projects. Do them together, and you may even realize you are still a child at heart.

The great thing about children is that they don't judge or criticize their creative endeavors or find a million excuses as to why they aren't capable of doing it well. They just do it. They do it because they love to create. They don't care if they color outside the lines or make a monster or creature that doesn't really exist or write a story that makes no sense. Children spend most of their time in the present, not yet torn between the agony of past actions and the dread of future events.

Depriving anyone, adult or child, of the ability to be creative is a recipe for unhappiness, lack of fulfillment, lack of purpose, and a diminished sense of individuality. Open your child's eyes and mind to find new ways to create. Allowing inspiration and creativity to become a part of their lives are gifts they can carry with them into adulthood.

## THE ART OF CREATION

It is your birthright to express who you are. You do this best through your creative endeavors. They are your individual stamp on the world and make you unique. Every time you fight the urge to be creative, you suppress a powerful and ancient desire to take nothingness and turn it into somethingness. That begins in the mind with a simple "aha" moment, one that comes from becoming present to the flow of life.

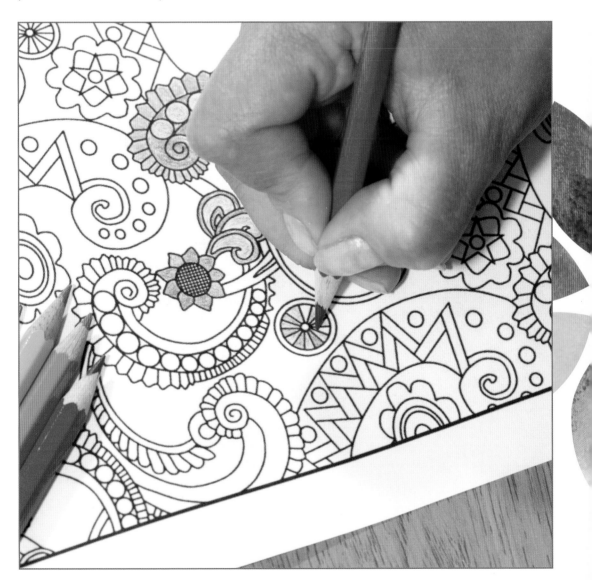

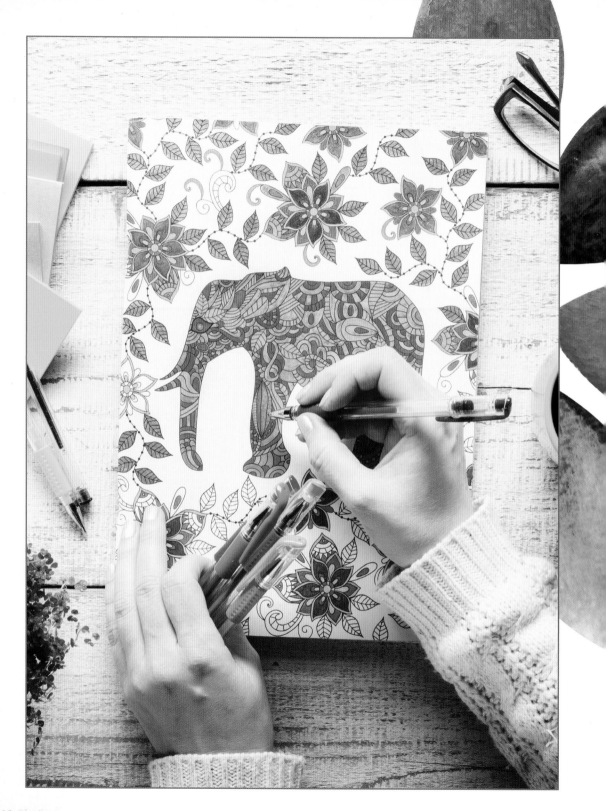